Gun Violence

STUDIES IN CRIME AND PUBLIC POLICY
Michael Tonry and Norval Morris, *General Editors*

Police for the Future
David H. Bayley

Incapacitation: Penal Confinement and the Restraint of Crime
Franklin E. Zimring and Gordon Hawkins

The American Street Gang: Its Nature, Prevalence, and Control
Malcolm W. Klein

Sentencing Matters
Michael Tonry

The Habits of Legality: Criminal Justice and the Rule of Law
Francis A. Allen

Chinatown Gangs: Extortion, Enterprise, and Ethnicity
Ko-lin Chin

Responding to Troubled Youth
Cheryl L. Maxson and Malcolm W. Klein

Making Crime Pay: Law and Order in Contemporary American Politics
Katherine Beckett

Community Policing, Chicago Style
Wesley G. Skogan and Susan M. Hartnett

Crime Is Not the Problem: Lethal Violence in America
Franklin E. Zimring and Gordon Hawkins

Hate Crimes: Criminal Law & Identity Politics
James B. Jacobs and Kimberly Potter

Politics, Punishment, and Populism
Lord Windlesham

American Youth Violence
Franklin E. Zimring

Bad Kids: Race and the Transformation of the Juvenile Court
Barry C. Feld

Punishment, Communication, and Community
R. A. Duff

Punishment and Democracy: Three Strikes and You're Out in California
Franklin E. Zimring, Gordon Hawkins, and Sam Kamin

Gun Violence: The Real Costs
Philip J. Cook and Jens Ludwig

Gun VIOLENCE _____

the real costs

Philip J. Cook
Jens Ludwig

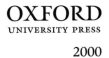

OXFORD
UNIVERSITY PRESS

2000

OXFORD

UNIVERSITY PRESS

Oxford   New York

Athens   Auckland   Bangkok   Bogotá   Buenos Aires   Calcutta
Cape Town   Chennai   Dar es Salaam   Delhi   Florence   Hong Kong   Istanbul
Karachi   Kuala Lumpur   Madrid   Melbourne   Mexico City   Mumbai
Nairobi   Paris   São Paulo   Shanghai   Singapore   Taipei   Tokyo   Toronto   Warsaw

and associated companies in
Berlin   Ibadan

Published by Oxford University Press, Inc.
198 Madison Avenue, New York, New York 10016

Oxford is a registered trademark of Oxford University Press.

Library of Congress Cataloging-in-Publication Data
Cook, Philip J., 1946–
Gun violence: the real costs / Philip J. Cook and Jens Ludwig.
p. cm — (Studies in crime and public policy)
Includes bibliographical references and index.
ISBN 0-19-513793-0
1. Gun control—United States—Costs.
2. Violent crimes—United States—Prevention.
I. Ludwig, Jens.   II. Title. III. Series.
HV7436.C663   2000
364.15'0973—dc21   00-028556

C717g

1 2 3 4 5 6 7 8 9

Printed in the United States of America
on acid-free paper

For Cammie and Brian
P.J.C.

For Almuth, Gunter, Abi, and Liz.
J.L.

Preface

The urge to put a dollar value on life and limb comes naturally to economists. To normal people, however, this may seem unnecessary and even a bit perverse. What's the point? In particular, they may question why we have gone to the trouble of writing an entire book that tries to measure the effect of gunshot injuries and deaths on our standard of living. Just how is it helpful to translate fear, pain, disability, and early death into the same metric as we ordinarily use in measuring the consumption of food, shelter, and transportation?

We have two answers. The first is that putting a monetary value on gun violence is useful in laying claim to public attention. If gun violence is to "compete" effectively in the public forum with other problems—highway deaths, breast cancer, air pollution, failing schools—then gun violence needs a dollar-cost number, simply because such numbers have become a standard item in policy discourse. Our estimate, that gun violence costs something on the order of $100 billion each year, turns out to be large enough to support a case for greater attention and effort.

Our second answer is more substantive. In conducting our research for this project, we have found that the economic-cost framework provides a different and more useful understanding of the problem than does the usual array of public-health statistics. Reporting 30,000 deaths and 80,000 serious injuries places the focus on the victims and may lead to an assessment of how "they" are different from the rest of us. It is all too easy to discount the suicides as mentally ill, the assault victims as careless or worse. But viewed from the economic perspective, the focus becomes far wider, encompassing not just actual victims, but potential victims and those who are linked to those potential victims by family, friendship, or finances. In short, most all of us bear some part of the costs of gun violence, in myriad ways: waiting in line to pass through airport security; buying a transparent book bag for school aged children to meet their school's post-Columbine regulations; paying taxes for the protection of public officials, for urban renewal projects in areas devastated by gun violence, for subsidizing an urban trauma center; living in fear that one's children may be injured by a stray bullet or that a despondent relative would get her hands on a gun. And no one is entirely safe from becoming a victim themselves.

The goal is thus to document how gun violence reduces the quality of life for everyone in America. Recasting the problem in this way will, we hope, help inform the "Great American Gun War" to take us past symbolic politics to a direct engagement with the costs and benefits of alternative policies. This shift in emphasis helps focus sustained attention on those interventions that hold promise for reducing gun violence and may pay for themselves.

We can briefly outline the presentation. Chapter 1 provides a broad overview of our main arguments and conclusions, while subsequent chapters develop these points in greater detail. Chapter 2 describes statistical patterns of gun violence in America. Assaults and unintentional shootings are concentrated among young Hispanics and especially African Americans, while suicide rates tend to increase in late middle age and be higher for whites than minorities. All types of gun violence fall disproportionately on the poor and overwhelmingly on males rather than females, but no group is entirely spared.

Of course, guns are not the only instruments of violence; other weapons account for a third of homicides and 40% of suicides. But our focus remains on guns so as to provide a basis for evaluating the array of policy measures that are targeted on reducing gun use in violence, rather than in reducing overall rates of violence. It is, in fact, the use of guns in violent crime that makes America unique among industrialized nations. As we document in Chapter 3, greater use of guns makes the problem of violence worse in America because guns are more lethal than the other weapons typically used in assaults and suicide attempts. The implication is that separating guns from violence saves lives.

Chapter 4 provides an accounting framework for monetizing the benefits of reducing gun violence. This is not a straightforward exercise, and the literature includes a variety of methods. In order to understand the different ways in which gun violence reduces the quality of life in America, we offer the image of a "vaccine" that would reduce the threat of gunshot injury; tracing through all of the ways in which the public would benefit helps highlight a number of costs that have been ignored in previous studies of this topic There would be less need for investments in prevention, avoidance, and harm reduction, both public and private, and less concern about being shot or losing a loved one or a neighbor to gunfire.

The traditional "Cost of Illness" framework used by public health researchers directs our attention to the medical costs and lost productivity associated with gunshot injuries. We look into these matters in Chapters 5 and 6, finding that these costs, while large in some absolute sense, are smaller than previous studies suggest and constitute only a modest share of the overall burden.

The greater costs of gun violence stem from the fact that all of us must live with the risk that we or someone we care about will be injured by gunfire. Chapter 7 lists some of the ways in which private citizens, businesses, and government agencies attempt to reduce the risk of gunshot injury. While we cannot quantify most of these adaptations, we show that they are likely to cost at least $5–10 billion per year, and probably far more.

To obtain a more comprehensive measure of costs, both subjective and tangible, we turn to a "contingent-valuation" survey that asks respondents what they would pay to reduce gun assaults. The results, presented in Chapter 8, suggest that the elimination of gun use in assault would be worth at least $80 billion per year. Elimination of unintentional shootings and gun suicides would be worth another $10–20 billion.

Chapter 9 then turns to a discussion of remedies. A variety of interventions hold promise for reducing misuse of guns, including traditional gun control measures (screening and registering buyers, prohibiting ownership by teenagers and felons), requiring gun manufacturers to incorporate safety features in their products, policing against illegal carrying, and threatening those who use guns in crime with longer prison sentences. The potential benefits of several such interventions, estimated using the results from previous chapters, are compared with estimated costs. Since some of these interventions arguably produce benefits in excess of costs, increasing their scope or intensity improves the overall standard of living in America.

Gun violence is a public health problem and a moral problem, but it is also a quality-of-life issue for all of us. We hope that the perspective offered in this book will provide some leverage in moving the policy debate toward a more reasoned response.

Durham, North Carolina   *P. J. C.*
Washington, D.C.   *J. L.*
July 2000

Acknowledgments

This book was made possible by a grant from the Joyce Foundation of Chicago and was written in part while Ludwig was a visiting scholar at the Northwestern University/University of Chicago Joint Center for Poverty Research. Our thanks to both organizations, though of course the views expressed herein in no way reflect those of our funders.

We are also grateful to the dedicated members of the advisory board for this project, including Arlene Greenspan, Steve Hargarten, David Hemenway, Arthur Kellermann, Jim Mercy, Will Manning, John Mullahy, Terry Richmond, William Schwab, and Daniel Webster. The contributions of this group have substantially improved the quality of our book.

We offer special thanks to Ted Miller and Bruce Lawrence, who collaborated with us on our study of the medical costs of gun violence. The results of our collaboration are presented in Chapter 5 and Appendix B, parts of which have also been published in the *Journal of the American Medical Association* (vol. 282, No. 5 [August 4, 1999]: 447–54). They have also provided us with a number of calculations and very useful comments for the other chapters as well.

Michael Tonry, Steve Levitt, and Dedi Felman read the entire draft manuscript and made a number of very useful suggestions. Other valuable comments were provided to us by Jeffrey Conte, Ted Gayer, Joel Huber, Helen Ladd, Jonathan Mathieu, Harold Pollack, Kurt Schwabe, Kerry Smith, Jon Vernick, Elizabeth Richardson Vigdor, Garen Wintemute, Mona Wright, and seminar participants at the 1998 meetings of the American Society of Criminology, the 1999 meetings of the American Economic Association, Duke University, and the University of North Carolina at Chapel Hill.

Access to the various data sources used in this book was facilitated by the generous assistance of Lee Annest, Mike DeVivo, Katherine Heck, Richard Linn, Ellen O'Brien, and Margaret Warner. We are also grateful to the Johns Hopkins Center for Gun Policy and Research and the National Opinion Research Center at the University of Chicago, particularly Steve Teret, Alma Kuby, and Tom Smith, for allowing us to include questions on their annual gun survey and working with us to develop the survey items themselves. The other members of our research team at Duke, Georgetown, and Northwestern universities— Christina Clark, Heath Einstein, Jessica Lucas, Bob Malme, Ike McFarlin, Josh Pinkston, Esperanza Ross, and Jennifer Sturiale—provided outstanding research assistance that went far beyond the call of duty.

Judy Cook and Elizabeth Scott displayed (nearly) endless patience during the writing of the book and provided us with much-needed support and good humor.

Finally, we owe a unique debt to our supporters at the Joyce Foundation. Roseanna Ander has been an unflagging source of ideas and enthusiasm; without her, the book would never have been finished. Of course, the book would never have begun without the encouragement of Debby Leff, at the time the president of the Joyce Foundation, and the inspiration of Mary O'Connell. Lore has it that Mary came up with the idea for a project on the costs of gun violence during a staff meeting at the Joyce Foundation's headquarters several years ago, in response to a question by Debby about what kind of research might really move gun policy forward in America. This book, then, is the ultimate result of Mary's idea, combined with the well-known natural law that no one says no to Debby Leff. For getting us started, and for their assistance throughout, we are enormously grateful to them both.

Contents

Gun Violence

1

Gun Violence and Life in America

At 11:21 A.M. on April 20, 1999, 18-year-old Eric Harris and 17-year-old Dylan Klebold entered Columbine High School in Littleton, Colorado, from the back parking lot carrying two sawed-off shotguns, a Hi-Point semiautomatic rifle, and a 9 millimeter Tech DC 9 semi-automatic pistol with a high-capacity magazine.[1] The two students had earlier hidden at least 30 pipe bombs throughout the school for use in the attack[2] and had planted a 25-pound propane bomb in the school's kitchen.[3] They then proceeded to open fire, shooting 35 people before the end of lunch hour. By three in the afternoon, local police had finally evacuated the building and started their search for the gunmen, both of whom were found in the school library, dead of self-inflicted gunshot wounds.[4] Among the 13 other victims who died were 48-year-old Dave Sanders, a popular teacher who was shot twice in the chest while leading others to safety, and Daniel Rohrbough, a 15-year-old freshman who was shot while holding an exit door open for other students and was, as the *New York Times* reported, "last seen alive, running, screaming for his mother."[5] The family of Lauren Townsend, a senior and member of the National Honor Society, received a letter offering her a college scholarship the day of her funeral.[6]

It is difficult to overstate the effects that this tragedy has had on the residents of Littleton. The Columbine High School students' lives and those of their friends and families will never be the same. And the shock wave from these shootings has reverberated throughout Colorado. The mother of a high school student reports that up to that point, "I had total blind faith in the schools, but I am not going to play Russian roulette with her life. I just can't do it. She thinks about where she'd run and how she'd get out of her school if it happened to her. How do you study and concentrate like that?" Similar sentiments by other parents have led to a fourfold increase in the number of calls received by the Christian Home Educators of Colorado, a home-schooling organization.[7]

The Littleton shootings followed a string of similar, though more limited attacks by students at schools in Jonesboro, Arkansas (March 1998), West Paducah, Kentucky (December 1997), and Pearl, Mississippi (October 1997). They have touched parents and students across the country. After Littleton, one teacher in a Virginia public school with many low-income students noted, "It may be hard for so-called safe communities to accept the fact that their children can inflict as much mayhem as, and maybe more than, those from less privileged environments and to take the tough steps that schools like mine have learned are the price of protection."[8]

Metal detectors, security personnel, and other measures that had once been largely confined to big cities are now in schools across the country. Many principals and other school personnel spent the summer of 1999 worried primarily about student safety:

> In dozens of locales as disparate as Pittsburgh and Palm Beach County, SWAT teams have spent the summer learning the layouts of high schools and conducting drills involving mock hostage-taking. Many students returning to school will find metal detectors and armed security guards at the doors, while others will have to trade their canvas backpacks for see-through bags designed to make it harder to conceal a weapon. . . . In Allen, Texas, a suburb of Dallas that cut back its class schedule last spring after a series of bomb threats, officials are spending $1 million to bring in metal detectors, surveillance cameras and a new security force, and are requiring students to wear identification badges.[9]

The Lessons of Littleton

The Littleton tragedy highlights several lessons that are important for addressing the problem of gun violence in America. First is the key role of technology. There have been endless commentaries on what could possibly have driven Harris and Klebold, sons of prosperous families with seemingly bright futures, to plan and execute the mass killing of their classmates and teachers. The suggestions range from the sterility of life in upscale subdivisions to the violent fantasies encouraged by television and computer games to general societal permissiveness. Whatever the merits of these various perspectives, one feature of this attack cannot be ignored: Harris and Klebold, like the other student killers before them, used guns to accomplish their grim purpose. They also tried, unsuccessfully, to use bombs, but without guns, the enterprise would have been unthinkable.

Of course, guns are not necessary to perpetrate more ordinary violence, whether in schools or homes or on the street. Knives, fists, and clubs are far more common. The importance of guns in routine fights and robberies is that they intensify violence, increasing the likelihood of death. Because guns increase the scope and lethality of violence, keeping them away from violent encounters is a vital public goal. This goal is distinct from the goal of reducing overall violence rates. Gun-oriented policies, if they are successful, may save lives even if assault and robbery rates stay at current levels.

A second lesson is that the consequences of Littleton and the other school shootings extend well beyond the injuries and loss of life. These tragedies created a new arena for worry, a violent scenario that parents and principals everywhere could not ignore. The anguish of the victims and their families and friends was just the beginning—throughout America the emotional response to the shootings engendered a demand for prevention and protection efforts.

Third, in aggregate these efforts to repair the damage to peace of mind are not cheap. The effort to prevent subsequent shootings has greatly added to the costs of the shootings themselves. That is, in assessing the comprehensive costs of gun violence in schools, we must include the direct burden created by the threat and the indirect burden on parents and children who are complying with the new rules, not to mention the taxpayers who are paying for the extra protection.

Fourth, in the costly pursuit of safety, it's possible to err on the side of "too much." While many schools responded to the Littleton shootings by substantially changing their security practices, others have rejected the use of metal detectors and similar measures as "an affront to educational openness."[10] One superintendent from Massachusetts said "We don't want to create an image of a police state, and we don't want dogs sniffing around," while the Los Angeles public schools decided against screening every student because of the loss in class time that would result.[11] The trade-off appears in the private sector as well: As one bank president said, "you don't want to have so much security that you inconvenience your customers."[12]

Systematic evaluation of policies to reduce gun violence thus requires that the costs on both sides be weighed and compared. But it is more common in debates over gun-oriented policies that the two sides talk past each other. Consider, for example, the use of aggressive police patrols against illegal gun carrying in New York. Mayor Rudolph Guiliani supports these patrols, arguing that they may well have contributed to the reduction in gun crime in the city. Opponents such as the Reverend Al Sharpton argue that the patrols should be ended in light of the inconvenience to large numbers of innocent and predominantly minority citizens. But presumably most observers will synthesize the two arguments and recognize that police patrols against illegal gun carrying involve both benefits and costs. In the absence of more information about the relative importance of each, members of the public are left to form their own opinions on the basis of other things, such as which spokesperson has the less unpleasant personality.

A More Comprehensive Perspective

To the extent that data rather than rhetoric are brought to bear in public discourse on gun problems, they consist of counts of injuries and deaths, rather than broader measures of effects on society and standards of living. Of course the immediate damage guns do in assaults, homicides, unintentional shootings, and suicides, amounting to more than a million deaths since 1965 and about three times that number of injuries, cannot be denied. Indeed, in considering the potential benefits of sentencing enhancements for gun use in crime, a ban on particularly dangerous types of guns, or more stringent regulation of gun commerce, the first question must be whether that policy will save lives and increase public safety. But even if the answer is yes, then there remains a second, more subtle question—what is the value of this increase in public safety, and how does it compare with the costs of the program?

The first question is challenging enough and produces any number of skirmishes among analysts. A case in point concerns the consequences of putting more guns on the street by easing restrictions on carrying a concealed weapon. The claim that gun-toting citizens will deter homicidal assaults contends with the claim that more guns on the street will simply escalate the "arms race." There is evidence on both sides, though in our judgment these policies have likely had little effect either way.

For other policies, such as sentencing enhancements for gun use in crime, the evidence of effectiveness is more clear cut. But knowing that a policy of this sort saves lives isn't enough for setting public policy, given the considerable costs of increasing our society's already high rate of incarceration.

The effort to place a value on increased safety expands the discussion. As in the Littleton example, the cost of gun violence is not limited to the immediate damage but has broad consequences for peace of mind, private investment in protection and avoidance, and the expenditure of tax revenues. With this broader perspective comes a surprising answer to the question of whose problem this is: While gun assaults and unintentional injuries are concentrated to a remarkable degree among a narrow demographic slice of the population—younger black or Hispanic men—the rest of the population is by no means immune. And in seeking to reduce our vulnerability, or paying our share of the public bill for responding to violence, the burden is widely shared.

This more comprehensive approach, defining gun violence as, in effect, a tax on our standard of living as well as a public health or crime issue, may help in the effort to create and sustain public attention on the problem. Too often, gun policies are adopted in response to highly publicized shootings.[13] The tendency is to focus on preventing similar events in the future, rather than on those policies that hold the most promise for reducing gunshot injuries over the long run. For example, because some of the weapons used in the Columbine school shootings were obtained from a gun show, a number of proposals have been made to regulate gun sales at gun shows—even though only a very small share of teens and convicted criminals obtain their firearms from this source. Scarce public attention and government resources are thus diverted toward programs that have narrow scope. Documenting the ongoing shared costs of gun violence may provide a more broad-gauged perspective on policymaking.

The Benefits of Reducing Gun Violence

Can we assign a monetary value to a human life, or to the suffering of someone who has been paralyzed by a gunshot wound, or to the effects of such injuries on the lives of family and friends? As difficult and unpleasant as this task may seem, the fact is that the courts regularly place a price on life and limb in setting damages for personal-injury suits; more to the point, legislatures and regulatory agencies are routinely required to decide how much an increment in safety is worth. When Congress established a national speed limit of 55 in 1974, the highway fatality rate dropped dramatically.[14] But much of the public, including the commercial trucking interests, eventually demanded a return to higher speed limits despite the likely increase in fatalities that would result, and Congress complied. Individual consumers are also forced to make decisions in the face of what might be thought of as a "quantity-quality" trade-off for our lives. Should we spend extra to obtain a car with dual air bags or antilock breaks, or save the money for a cruise in the Bahamas? Is that job cleaning windows on the exterior of the Empire State Building worth the extra pay? Should we pay an extra $10,000 to buy a house that is farther away from the local nuclear plant? And so forth.

To be clear, policymakers and private citizens are making judgments about the value of *ex ante* reductions in the risk of injury, before the identity of those who will be injured is known. While most people would give up much of their net worth to save themselves or a loved one from certain death, their willingness to pay for small reductions in the risk of death is more limited. It is the summation of what people will pay for small reductions in the probability of death that defines what is known as the "value of a statistical life," with values defined similarly for statistical injuries and other health hazards. If each person in a community of 100,000 is willing to pay $50 to reduce the number of injury deaths in that community by one per year, then the value of a statistical life to these residents equals $5 million.

What people will pay to reduce the risk of gunshot injury will presumably depend on how it affects them, their families, and their communities. Sometimes the monetary value of greater safety comes right off a spreadsheet. For example, the sharp declines in the rate of violent crime during the 1990s have brought windfall gains in property values to many property owners in urban neighborhoods. But most of what's at stake here are intangible commodities not traded in the marketplace— freedom from the threat of gun violence, relief from the necessity of taking steps to reduce the threat.

The most straightforward way to determine what people will pay to reduce gun violence is to ask them. When 1,200 American adults were asked such a question in 1998 by the National Opinion Research Center (NORC) at the University of Chicago, the average household was willing to pay around $240 per year to reduce gun crime by 30% in their community. Multiplying by the total number of households in the United States implies that a 30% reduction in gun assaults is worth nearly $24 billion, or approximately $1 million per gunshot injury. Extrapolating from that, we find the total cost of gunshot injuries from crime is about $80 billion per year.

Many economists (and other people as well) are understandably dubious about how seriously to take responses to surveys, particularly when they relate to what respondents would hypothetically be willing to pay for government programs (rather than for items with which they may have more direct knowledge). Nevertheless, the results of this survey imply a value per statistical life that is remarkably consistent with those derived from studies of actual behavior in other contexts.[15] Further, an extra $240 per year to reduce gun assaults by 30% does not seem unreasonable compared with the $1,800 that crime-prevention efforts cost the average American household each year,[16] especially since people's fear of crime seems to be motivated largely by the fear of *violent* crime.[17]

Moreover, the use of survey data is preferable to the main alternative, which is to extrapolate the value of what people would pay to reduce gun violence from the implied value of improved safety as revealed in workplace and other settings. On the one hand, a large percentage of gunshot victims are engaged in highly risky activity and appear to place relatively little value on their own lives. On the other hand, the payment that people will require to accept riskier jobs only captures the value of improvements in personal safety and excludes some of the most important benefits from reducing gun violence, such as a diminished risk of injury to loved ones and reduced need for caution in everyday life.

However, our survey data cover only assault and homicide. To place a value on unintentional shootings or gun suicides, we do, with some trepidation, borrow numbers from other arenas. After adjusting for differences in age and risk between those at high risk of gunshot injury and the population as a whole, our calculations suggest that the elimination of unintentional gunshot injuries and gun suicides is probably worth as much as

$20 billion per year. Adding these estimates to those obtained from our survey data for gun assaults suggests that the annual costs of gun violence are on the order of $100 billion.

These results serve to highlight the importance of using the right accounting framework. Traditionally, policymakers have focused on a framework known as the "cost of illness" method, which in practice is the sum of victims' medical expenses (and other "direct costs" of injuries) and the value of their lost earnings. In spirit, this method borrows from national-product accounting and ignores most of what is captured in the willingness-to-pay approach: the subjective value of safety, concern about others' welfare, and the costs of prevention and avoidance. The bottom line is that medical expenses and lost productivity make up very little of the societal burden of gun violence.

Policy Evaluation

With more than 200 million guns in private hands,[18] many people are understandably skeptical about the ability of public policy to reduce the burden of gun violence. Yet there are interventions that hold promise in reducing the volume of gunshot injuries in America and may have benefits that exceed the costs.

Efforts to keep guns away from those deemed at high risk for misusing them has been an important goal of gun policy, though these policies have been criticized for their potentially negative effects on the ability of citizens to defend themselves. For example, James Q. Wilson has argued that "Guns are almost certainly contributors to the lethality of American violence, but there is no politically or legally feasible way to reduce the stock of guns now in private possession to the point that their availability to criminals would be much affected. . . . And even if there were, law-abiding people would lose a means of protecting themselves long before criminals lost a means of attacking them."[19] Yet we believe that Wilson exaggerates the difficulty of discriminating between law-abiding adults, on the one hand,

and teenagers and criminals on the other. Restrictions on gun sales and background checks to enforce them have the potential to produce some increase in the effective price of guns to high-risk people, while imposing only minor inconvenience to people outside of the disqualified groups.

In our view, perhaps the top priority for gun policy is to close the gaping loophole in the current regulatory system, which exempts private sales of used guns from the background-check requirements imposed on licensed gun dealers. In order to regulate these private sales, law-enforcement authorities must be able to hold owners accountable for their firearms. Requiring that all transfers be channeled through federally licensed dealers, and holding owners responsible for misuse of their guns, would be a good start. This requirement would affect about 2 million gun transfers each year, each of which would be required to go through a dealer. If the extra hassle to the seller, buyer, and dealer is worth a combined $100 worth of their time, then by our calculation the requirement is worthwhile if it prevents only 200 gunshot injuries per year.

The regulation of firearms as consumer products also has the potential to reduce gun misuse by improving gun design. The most promising new option in design is to "personalize" guns, thereby preventing them from being fired by persons other than the authorized owner. This technology—really a variety of different technological options—holds some promise for saving lives by making guns inoperable to despondent teenagers, curious children, or others (including burglars) who acquire guns in unauthorized fashion. While it is too soon to evaluate the net effect on public health, since even modest beneficial effects can make personalized gun technology worthwhile, we believe this technology is likely to provide considerable gains to society.

More traditional law-enforcement activities can also have a substantial effect in reducing criminal gun misuse. One demonstration found that less than $200,000 in extra funding for targeted police patrols against illegal gun carrying may have substantially reduced the number of gunshot injuries in the impacted neighborhoods. Our estimates suggest that the value to society from this change in gun violence is on the order of $20 to $100 million. Similarly, sentence enhancements for the use of guns in crime may also produce benefits far in excess of costs.

In sum, there are a variety of programs to reduce gun violence that enjoy widespread popular support, have little effect on the ability of most private citizens to keep guns for personal use, and have benefits that exceed costs. The last point is easy to justify once we recognize the magnitude of the burden that the threat of gun injuries imposes on our society.

2

Victimization Risks

The burden that gun violence imposes on our society can be described in a variety of ways. In subsequent chapters, we turn to the task of expressing this burden in dollar terms, but we begin with the more familiar indicators of the impact on public health.

Gun violence causes a large number of injuries each year, many of them fatal. The magnitudes, trends, and distribution of these injuries form the statistical backdrop to the public debate over gun policy. And they also provide some insight into why the case for more regulation of gun design, marketing, and possession has been difficult to make in the political arena. Before the mass shooting at Columbine High, it was all too easy for middle-class Americans to see gun injuries as someone else's problem.

The body count is daunting. In 1997, over 32,000 Americans died of gunshot wounds—more than died from AIDS or liver disease in that year, and in the same ballpark with motor-vehicle crashes (42,000). Since 1965 more than *one million* people have been shot and killed, more than the number of Americans killed in all foreign wars combined during the twentieth century (617,000). Our firearms death rate is not the highest in the world—Columbia's, for example, is higher—but exceeds that of any other developed nation by a wide margin.

Gunshot fatalities impose a disproportionate public-health impact because so many of the victims are young. A measure that takes account of that fact is "years of potential life lost before the age of 65" (YPLL-65). Firearms injury was ranked

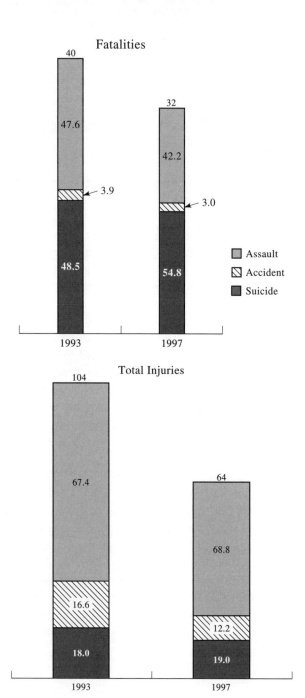

number four in YPLL-65 during the early 1990s, behind only unintentional injury, cancer, and heart disease.[1] Actually the Vital Statistics do not usually group gun deaths together; instead they are found with the homicides and suicides (both of which have guns as the agent in the majority of cases) and unintentional deaths. Homicide and suicide each rank among the top four causes of death for youths age 10–34.[2]

Trends

The all-time peak in the number of Americans killed or injured by gunshot in peacetime occurred in 1993. The total was 39,595 deaths and 131,000 injuries requiring medical treatment. By 1997, these totals had dropped to 32,436 deaths and just 81,000 injuries, and early reports indicate further progress in 1998 and 1999. (See Table A1 in Appendix A for details.) As shown in Figure 2.1, gun homicide and accidents dropped much farther proportionately than did suicide during this interval.

Figure 2.1 also provides other information on the relative importance of the different circumstances. In 1997, unintentional shootings accounted for just 3% of the fatalities; suicides account for 55% and homicides for the remaining 48%. This distribution is quite different when nonfatal injuries are included, for the simple reason that suicide attempts with a gun are almost always fatal (the "case fatality rate" is over 80%), while only 7% of unintentional shootings are fatal. Assaults are more numerous than unintentional shootings and far less lethal (with a case fatality rate of 17%) than suicide. Thus while half or more of fatalities are suicide, the great majority of gunshot

Figure 2.1. Gun Related Fatalities and Injuries, 1993 and 1997, Percentage Distribution by Circumstance. *Note*: The number of victims is shown at the top of each bar, in thousands, and the area of each bar is proportional to that count. *Top*: Data provided by the Vital Statistics, National Center for Health Statistics. *Bottom*: Data provided by the Vital Statistics, National Center for Health Statistics, and the National Electronic Injury Surveillance System, Centers for Disease Control and Prevention.

cases that show up in the emergency departments and trauma centers are the result of criminal assault.

Figure 2.2 provides trend information for the period following World War 2, depicting death rates by five-year interval since 1950. The bottom half of the figure shows that suicide rates per 100,000 have been remarkably steady during the postwar period: there was a modest upward trend from 10.2 in 1955 to 12.5 in 1975, and since then rates have been flat. What has changed during this period has been the *means* of committing suicide. Guns accounted for just 43% of suicides in 1950 but had climbed to 50% in 1970 and nearly 60% during the 1990s.

As shown in the top half of Figure 2.2, homicide rates have been far more variable and indeed have undergone the greatest fluctuations of any of the leading causes of death. Homicide with guns has been particularly volatile. Both gun and nongun homicide rates peaked in 1980, with gun homicide three times as high as in 1955.[3] The decline since 1993 has taken rates down to a level last seen in the mid-1960s.

The sharp increase in homicide and suicide rates during the period 1965–1980 is all the more noteworthy given what was happening with other causes of trauma deaths during this period. Figure 2.3 depicts the secular decline in motor vehicle death rates that began in 1970, coupled with the much longer and steeper decline in the death rate due to all other kinds of unintentional injury. Thus the trends in intentional killings bucked the overall trend toward a safer society.

What is missing from these pictures is a sense of the profound changes in demographic patterns of homicide that occurred during the later part of this time period. From 1985 until 1993, there was a great epidemic of gun violence, concentrated in the group that has always borne the heaviest load of gun violence: young Hispanic and especially African American males. The homicide victimization rate for black males age 13–17 tripled during this period, while this rate doubled for those 18–24. All of this increase was due to gun use. Occurring during a time when homicide rates for older people were actually declining, the epidemic concentrated homicide still further on minority youths.[4]

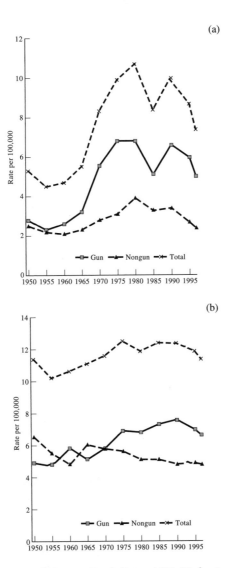

Figure 2.2. Gun and Nongun Death Rates, 1950–97, by 5-year Interval:
a Homicide Rates; *b* Suicide Rates. *a*: Data provided by the Vital
Statistics, National Center for Health Statistics. *b*: Data provided by the
Vital Statistics, National Center for Health Statistics.

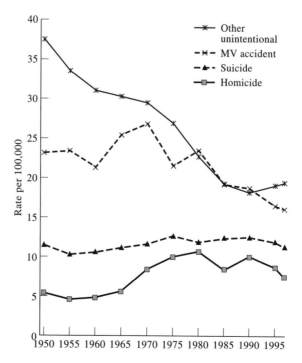

Figure 2.3. Injury-Death Rates, 1950–97, by 5 year Interval. Data provided by the Vital Statistics, National Center for Health Statistics.

The usual explanation for this epidemic is in terms of the introduction of crack cocaine into one city after another during the 1980s. The new illicit markets provided young people in urban areas with the means and the motivation to arm themselves in a high-conflict situation, with disastrous results.[5] Since 1993, as crack markets have matured and stabilized, homicide rates have declined for this group as dramatically as they increased before.

The age profile of suicide has also shifted during the last two decades. There has been a strong secular trend upward in adolescent suicide with guns, catching them up to the victimization rates of adults. During the 1980s, there was a sharp increase at the other end of the age spectrum; those 75 and over experienced a sharp increase in suicide that has placed that group's suicide rate well above all others.[6]

The Concentration of Gun Violence

The victims of gun violence are far from a cross section of the American public. Particularly in the case of homicide and assault, young minority males, and those with criminal records, are greatly overrepresented. For suicide, the demographic concentration is not as great, but the less visible dimensions—mental illness and chronic disease—tend to distinguish suicides from the rest of the population. These patterns no doubt contribute to marginalizing the gun problem in the public agenda.

Many public health problems take a particularly severe toll on those with low socioeconomic status, and gun violence is no exception. Documenting the socioeconomic patterns of death has only recently become possible, thanks to the expansion beginning in 1989 of the information collected in the Vital Statistics census of deaths. Another source of data on the victims of fatal gunshot injuries comes from the 1993 National Mortality Followback Survey (NMFS), which obtained more detailed sociodemographic information for a sample of about 23,000 decedents from next-of-kin surveys (see Appendix A for details).

In Tables A2 through A7 of Appendix A, we report mortality rates for different population subgroups defined by gender, age, race / ethnicity, educational attainment, employment, and family income from all sources. Here we summarize the results in a series of bar charts.

Gun Homicides

Figure 2.4 depicts homicide patterns for males in 1996, demonstrating the importance of age and race particularly. For example, the gun homicide rate for Hispanic men ages 18–29 equals 38.5 per 100,000, around seven times the rate for white men of the same age; the gun homicide rate for black men 18–

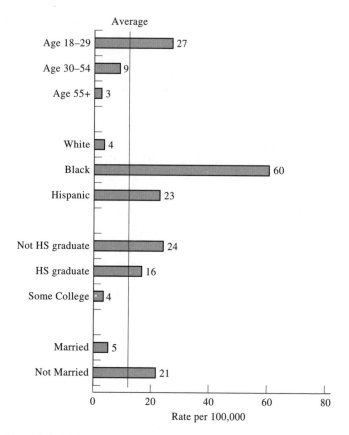

Figure 2.4. Male Homicide Victimization Rates, 1996. Data provided by the 1996 Vital Statistics, National Center for Health Statistics.

29 is an astonishing 133.5 per 100,000, around 25 times the rate for whites. Homicide patterns for women are similar but at a much lower level—about 80% of all homicide victims are male.

It is of interest to know how much of those large differences by race can be accounted for by group differences in education and marital status. Blacks in particular are less likely to enjoy the protective effect of a high school degree or a marriage license. As it turns out, the gaps appear large even when we limit the comparison to those who are similarly situated: among married high-school graduates age 18–29, for example, the victimization rates are 2.6 (whites), 16.1 (Hispanics), and 75.8 (blacks).[7]

In addition to the demographic factors explored here, behavior is also a strong predictor of homicide victimization. In particular, criminal involvement is a major risk factor for homicide. A study of all homicide victims ages 21 and younger in Boston between 1990 and 1994 found that three-quarters had prior criminal records.[8] William Schwab and his colleagues at the University of Pennsylvania found that in Philadelphia the proportion of gun homicide victims with prior criminal records increased from 73% in 1985 to 84% in 1990 and by 1996 was fully 93%.[9] And data from the Virginia Department of Justice for adolescents in Richmond show that the risk of gunshot injury is 22 times higher for males who are involved in crime than those who aren't.[10]

Gun Suicides

Suicide patterns are similar to homicide with respect to sex but not race or age. Indeed, suicide rates are highest among the elderly population in America, and generally higher for whites than other groups.[11] While women attempt suicide around three times as often as men, suicide fatalities among men outnumber those for women by four to one, and the gap is still larger for gun suicide.[12] As in the case of homicide, marriage and education appear to have some protective effect. Figure 2.5 tells this story.

While many suicide attempts by young people involve alcohol and appear to be impulsive,[13] more than 90% of suicide victims suffer from some mental or addictive disorder. Psychiatrist Kay Redfield Jamison provides this summary: "The most common element in suicide is psychopathology, or mental illness; of the disparate mental illnesses, a relative few are particularly and powerfully bound to self-inflicted death: the mood disorders (depression and manic-depression), schizophrenia, borderline and antisocial personality disorders, alcoholism, and drug abuse."[14]

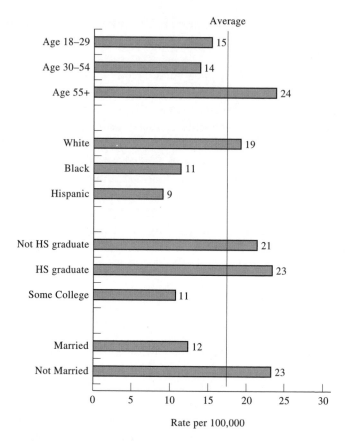

Figure 2.5. Male Suicide Victimization Rates, 1996. Data provided by the Vital Statistics, National Center for Health Services.

Impaired physical health also is associated with suicide risk, as we've found in exploring the NMFS data. The NMFS includes information on health prior to the victim's death, including whether the victim had spent time in a nursing home or hospice during the last year of life, suffered from a serious health problem,[15] required the use of a serious medical assistive device (such as dialysis equipment), or had trouble with even basic household chores during the year before death.

These data leave some doubt about the sequence of events—a few may have been hospitalized prior to death *because* they shot themselves and didn't die immediately. With that qualification in mind, we find that as many as 40% of all gun-suicide victims in 1993 suffered from poor health before they committed suicide (see details in Appendix A, Table A8). That seems quite large, but we don't know for sure how it compares with the population of the same age who did not commit suicide, since there are no comparable health-status measures available for the general population. However, we do have available various possible samples of the general population in the NMFS data. We chose victims of motor vehicle crashes as our comparison sample, limiting the analysis to those age 15 to 55. Victims of motor vehicle crashes may have been different from the general population in some ways, such as involvement in drinking and risky behavior, but we do not expect them to have been more or less burdened by medical impairment than others. As seen in Table 2.1, the proportion of gun-suicide victims who

Table 2.1

Poor Health for Firearm Suicide Victims vs. Other Fatalities

	Gun suicide victims, 15–55 years of age	Motor vehicle crash victims, 15–55 years of age
Indicators of poor health	Percent of Victims with Indicated Characteristic	
1. Victim ever lived in/admitted overnight to nursing home, hospice, or other health care facility	5.8	1.9
2. Victim had serious health problem[a]	9.8	5.2
3. Victim homebound last year of life	0.3	0.1
4. Victim required medical assistive device[b]	2.4	1.5

Table 2.1 *(Continued)*

Indicators of poor health	Gun suicide victims, 15–55 years of age	Motor vehicle crash victims, 15–55 years of age
	Percent of Victims with Indicated Characteristic	
5. Victim's family had "excessive" medical expenditures year before death[c]	1.1	1.7
6. Victim had difficulty with household chores year before death[d]	16.8	6.0
Proportion with poor health markers		
1 & 2	14.7	6.7
1, 2, & 3	14.9	6.7
1, 2, 3 & 4	15.7	7.7
1, 2, 3, 4, & 5	16.0	8.1
1, 2, 3, 4, 5, & 6	25.3	11.8

Notes: Estimates obtained from the 1993 National Mortality Followback Survey (NMFS), using the NMFS sampling weights to adjust for oversampling. Sample is constrained to those decedents who suffered their injuries in 1993, to eliminate cases in which poor health is a consequence of the lingering effects of an earlier injury that ultimately caused the death.

[a] Defined as those who have suffered a stroke, have Alzheimer's, dementia, senility, or some other organic brain impairment, cancer, or a lung illness (emphysema or bronchitis). We also include cirrhosis cases, though in practice no gunshot suicides had this disease.

[b] Victim required one of the following: infusion pump; shunt, catheter, tube, or surgically inserted access device in vein to allow for infusion of fluids, medication or intravenous feeding while living at home during last year of life; dialysis equipment; or oxygen or devices for breathing therapy.

[c] The NMFS provides information on the family's total out-of-pocket expenditures on medical care for the decedent during the year before death. It is not possible to determine how much of this spending was devoted to treatment for the injury that resulted in death versus other medical care during the year. Further, the NMFS does not identify total medical care spending from all sources. We assume that decedents whose families personally paid more than twice the average medical cost of a fatal gunshot suicide (as reported in Cook et al., 1999) were chronically ill.

[d] Defined as difficulty with the following activities because of physical or mental illness: lifting objects weighing as much as 10 pounds; climbing a flight of stairs; walking a quarter mile; shopping for food; going outside of the home alone; light work around the home; preparing meals; managing money; getting around the home; eating; using the toilet; bathing or showering; and dressing.

were in poor health prior to their injury is about twice the rate observed for victims of motor vehicle accidents. We conclude that chronic physical-health problems are an important risk factor for suicide.

Unintentional Shootings

Unintentional shootings form a rather small and dwindling portion of the total. Sociodemographic patterns for unintentional gunshot injuries reinforce the patterns we have already seen. One-third of all victims of fatal unintentional shootings in the United States are under the age of 20, and nearly 60% are under the age of 30.[16] As with gun homicides and suicides, the large majority of victims (nearly 90%) are male.[17] Unintentional shootings follow the same pattern across socioeconomic strata as homicides and suicides, with rates that are consistently higher for those of lower education or income.

The Reach of Gun Violence

While gun violence is highly concentrated in the United States, our rates of gun violence are so high that even people who are at relatively low risk by American standards are "at risk" by international standards. For example, data from 1996 suggests that the gun-homicide rate for married American adults 30 and older who have four-year college degrees is around 1.1 per 100,000.[18] By comparison, this rate is almost identical to the overall homicide rate in the Netherlands and Greece, and higher than the homicide rates in Norway, Ireland, and Spain.[19]

The lesson of these statistics, like that of the Littleton shootings, is that no one is immune to gun violence in America.

3

How Guns Matter

On December 8, 1980, Mark Chapman approached John Lennon outside his apartment building in New York City, pulled a cheap five-shot revolver, and shot him. Lennon died within minutes on his way to the hospital.[1] Afterward Chapman told the police, "Most of me didn't want to do it, but a little of me did. I couldn't help myself."[2] In December 1999, another former Beatle, George Harrison, was attacked in his mansion outside of London by a "fan," this one wielding a knife. Harrison was stabbed in the chest but not seriously injured. Together with his wife, he was able to fight off the assailant and hand him over to the police when they arrived on the scene.[3] The contrasting outcomes of these attacks help tell a larger story.

Among the prosperous nations of the world, the United States is distinctive not so much because of its high volume of violent crimes but because of the relatively high percentage of these crimes that involve guns, and the immediate consequence of that fact—a homicide rate far in excess of any other developed nation. Guns *intensify* violence. And for that reason it is a worthy goal of public policy to keep guns out of violent encounters.

This goal is to be distinguished from the quest to reduce *overall* rates of violence, which requires a very different set of interventions. A number of criminal-justice interventions and social programs show promise in this regard. Broad-based deterrence achieved through more police or stiffer prison sentences may work.[4] And the evidence on the crime-preventive effects of some social programs is quite promising: We would include intensive early-childhood interventions[5] and relocation of families of at-risk youths to low-poverty neighborhoods.[6] A variety of suicide-prevention programs are thought to be effective by mental health professionals.

In contrast, efforts to reduce the use of guns in violence focus on limiting the availability of guns to high-risk groups and the accessibility of guns in volatile situations. Examples that come readily to mind from recent public debates include mandating background checks on gun purchasers, banning small, easily concealed handguns, intensive patrolling against illegal gun carrying, and imposing stiffer sentences on those convicted of using a gun in crime. If such measures reduce gun misuse, they will save lives. Indeed, George Harrison may owe his life to the difficulty of obtaining a handgun in Britain. The regulation of gun access and use is thus a harm-reduction strategy, akin to installing air bags in motor vehicles.

Our interest in measuring the costs of gun violence stems largely from the need to evaluate programs designed to separate guns from violence. Understanding the benefits produced by such interventions is crucial for deciding how to balance this goal against other pressing social problems. Of particular importance is gaining some understanding of what happens in potentially violent encounters when guns are made less readily available. If the reduction in gun use resulting from a gun-oriented policy intervention tends to be coupled by an increase in nongun violence, then both changes must be considered in evaluating the net benefits of the program—it is the net effect on injury and death that matters.

How does, in fact, the reduction of gun misuse affect the volume and nature of violence? One possibility is that of "no replacement," where the elimination of guns results in the elimination of all those violent acts that would have been committed with guns. Other possibilities include "replacement with reduced harm," where gun killings are replaced one for one with less deadly assaults by other means, and "full replacement with equal harm," in which case the alternative weapons prove just as lethal as guns would have been. And some have argued that efforts to separate guns from violence may actually be counterproductive, by disarming law-abiding citizens who use guns for self-protection against criminal predators.

The available evidence suggests to us that for interpersonal violence the most likely scenario is that of "replacement with reduced harm," although the case for suicide is more ambiguous. Before turning to these matters, however, it is useful to set the stage by describing actual and proposed gun-oriented interventions.

Gun Controls and Other Gun-Oriented Policies

Consider the sequence of events that leads to a shooting. The assailant must acquire the gun, bring or carry it to the scene of the encounter, and then deploy it against the victim. Law-enforcement and regulatory agencies may intervene in any of these three areas. Here are some examples of where and how such interventions can be focused:

Acquisition
  Prohibit ownership by youths and criminals
  Regulate transactions
  Require secure storage
  Raise the excise tax on guns and ammunition
  Impose antitheft measures on dealers
  Conduct gun buy backs

Carry to Scene
  Ban concealed carrying or require a license
  Patrol against illicit carrying
  Ban small easily concealed guns
  Screen entrants at public buildings

Use in Crime
  Regulate gun design to reduce lethality
  Mandate sentence enhancements for gun use in crime

The restrictions on "Acquisition" are at the core of the gun-control debate, together with the product-design restrictions that show up in all three areas. For the most part, the objective in this first group of measures is to reduce gun use in crime by restricting supply and thus making it more difficult, time consuming, or costly for a violent individual to obtain a gun.

U.S. policies in this regard are weaker than in other prosperous nations—the United Kingdom, for example, banned the private ownership of all handguns in 1998, while it has never been possible for a private individual to obtain a handgun in Japan except under extraordinary circumstances.[7] U.S. policy is geared to preserving the legitimate uses of most types of guns for most people while restricting access for people and types of guns that are deemed unacceptably dangerous.

The federal Gun Control Act of 1968 established a regulatory framework for gun commerce with the intention of providing some insulation for states that opted for stricter regulations from more-lax states. In particular, mail-order firearms shipments may only be made to federally licensed dealers, and those dealers, who constitute the "primary" retail market, are required to keep records of shipments received as well as sales. The act also established a partial prohibition on gun possession, including a rather sizable swath of the U.S. population: those with a felony conviction or conviction for domestic violence or dishonorable discharge from the armed service; those under indictment; fugitives from justice; illegal aliens; users of illicit drugs; and those committed to a mental institution. Further, dealers are prohibited from selling a handgun to anyone under 21, or a long gun to anyone under 18. Dealers also face some restrictions in making sales to out-of-state residents, the idea being that people should not be able to circumvent their home-state laws by driving across the border.

The original method for enforcing the partial prohibition on possession was simply to require that people purchasing guns from licensed dealers show identification and sign a statement testifying that they did not fit into any of the prohibited categories. By 1980 almost half the states, including 64% of the population, had gone beyond federal requirements by requiring that police be given an opportunity to run a background check on handgun buyers.[8] In 1993, Congress finally followed suit, establishing a national requirement of this sort by enacting the Brady Law. The requirement of a background check now applies to sales of all guns by dealers.

As far back as 1934, federal law required that all machine guns be registered, and placed a heavy tax on transfers. More ordinary guns also are subject to federal excise taxes: 10% for handguns and 11% for long guns. And there are minor restrictions on what kinds of guns can be imported or sold in the United States. Some jurisdictions have more far-reaching restrictions; for example, Chicago (since 1982) and Washington D.C. (since 1976) have an outright ban on residents acquiring handguns.

States and localities have legislated restrictions on the carrying and use of weapons, a topic that we develop in greater detail below. And most states have special sentencing enhancements in place for criminals convicted of using a gun in crime.

As we write this there is a national debate, and also many local debates, over the proper regulation of guns. Determining the public value of additional regulations has never been more important.

The Volume of Violence

Guns are an essential element of some violent crimes. We don't see drive-by knifings or innocent bystanders killed by stray fists. Assassination attempts against well-defended public figures are most always with a gun. Guns are the weapon of choice for youths and office workers seeking to kill a large number of colleagues (although explosives may also come into play). A gun in such all-too-frequent scenarios is an essential element in perpetrating the crime.

But for the violent crimes that make up the usual fare of 911 calls, a gun is not required. Only around one-quarter of noncommercial robberies nationwide are committed with a gun,[9] and gun assaults are far outnumbered by fistfights and knifings. For such crimes, it is reasonable to suppose that if gun use were suppressed, gun threats and attacks would be replaced by assaults with other weapons.

There is little empirical evidence on the extent to which gun-oriented measures might lead to increases in nongun violent crime. One exception is a study of city robbery rates that concluded that the general availability of guns is closely linked to weapon choice by robbers, but has little relationship to the overall robbery rate. (Robbery is defined to include muggings, holdups, and other crimes where the victim is coerced into parting with valuables by threat or violence.) Among the 50 largest cities there exist large differences in gun ownership (10% of households in Boston, up to 50% in Phoenix and Denver) that were closely mirrored by the gun percentage in robbery. But gun prevalence did not appear to influence the overall (gun plus nongun) robbery rates in these cites.[10]

Similarly, Europeans' impression of the United States as a dangerous place to visit due to all the gun-wielding predators may well be justified, but with respect to nongun violence, it's a different story. Italy and Australia, for example, have overall robbery rates comparable to that in the United States, while Canada, Finland, and the Netherlands have comparable assault rates, despite these nations' far-lower gun-ownership rates.[11] Franklin Zimring and Gordon Hawkins make these and other international comparisons to support the conclusion suggested by the title of their book—*Crime Is Not The Problem*.[12] The distinctive "problem" for the United States is not the volume of violent crime here, but its deadliness.

Instrumentality

What difference does it make if violent people use knives or clubs instead of guns? Does the "instrument" matter in terms of harm done? One view of "instrumentality" is summarized in the old bumper strip, "Guns don't kill people, people kill people." In murder trials, the killer's motivation and state of mind are explored thoroughly, whereas the type of weapon is often treated as an incidental detail except as it relates to the motivation. The opposite hypothesis, that the weapon matters a great deal in determining whether an assault victim lives or dies, is summarized by the view of entertainer (and apparent gun-control advocate) Ozzy Osbourne: "I keep hearing this thing that guns don't kill people, but people kill people. If that's the case, why do we give people guns when they go to war? Why not just send the people?"[13] In fact, the evidence compels us to believe that the type of weapon does matter.

The evidence in support of the instrumentality effect begins with the simple observation that a gun, uniquely among commonly available weapons, provides an attacker with the ability to kill quickly, with little effort or risk to self. It is "the great equalizer" that conveys lethal power even to those who lack strength or determination. For those who do not have a sustained intent to kill, or who may become squeamish, it negates any need for the sort of bloody involvement required by a knife or bare hands. The robber may pull the trigger almost by accident, but that's enough. A gun can kill at a distance and poses a risk to all in the vicinity.

The statistics bear out the common sense of these observations. Robberies and assaults committed with guns are more likely to result in the victim's death than are similar violent crimes committed with other weapons. For example, the case-fatality rate for gun robbery is three times as high as for robberies with knives and ten times as high as for robberies with other weapons.[14] Similarly, in injuries resulting from criminal assault the case-fatality rate is closely linked to the type of weapon,[15] as is also the case for family violence.[16]

The pattern of weapon-related case-fatality rates does not *prove* that the type of weapon matters, since whether the assailant uses a gun or not is in part a reflection of his intent. Some have even argued that difference in intent is the entire explanation for the observed difference in lethality.[17] The ease of killing someone, as determined by the type of weapon available to the attacker, is, in this view, of no consequence for whether the victim does in fact die.

But this argument isn't plausible on the face of it and doesn't stand up to the evidence. The seminal studies of Franklin Zimring[18] provide a basis for concluding that there is actually a good deal of overlap between fatal and nonfatal attacks; even in the case of potentially deadly attacks, assailants commonly lack a clear or sustained intent to kill. Zimring's argument is that homicide is a by-product of violent crime. Although the law determines the seriousness of the crime by whether the victim lives or dies, that outcome is not a reliable guide to the assailant's intent or state of mind.

One logical implication of this perspective is that there should be a close link between the overall volume of gun violence and the number of murders, and so there is. One study demonstrated that the change in cities' robbery-murder rates from year to year is closely linked to the underlying gun-robbery rate: An increase of 1,000 gun robberies per year results on the average in an additional 0.48 additional murders, whereas an additional 1,000 robberies with other weapons resulted in an additional 0.14 murders.[19] The close statistical link between robbery and robbery murder, together with descriptive evidence on the two crimes,[20] appear to confirm the view that much robbery murder is a by-product of robbery (rather than an event resulting from a distinct set of circumstances and motivations).

In essence, we hold with a different slogan: "Guns don't kill people; they just make it real easy."[21] But this conclusion is under heavy attack from those who assert the great importance of guns in self-defense, a topic that requires separate attention.

Self-Defense

Guns have virtuous as well as vicious uses, and in particular provide some crime victims with the means to fend off their assailants. Further, knowing that gun ownership is widespread may affect a violent person's decision of whether and how to act when he has a beef or some notion of committing rape or robbery. These observations are hard to dispute. What *is* in dispute is the magnitude of these effects and their implications for public policy. How often do victims succeed in using a gun to avoid serious injury? To what extent does the private ownership of guns serve as a deterrent to violence?

These questions are relevant to our cost analysis because if using guns in self-defense is common, then policy interventions intended to separate guns from violence may have the perverse effect of increasing the amount of violence, and in some cases making it more harmful. Our working assumption (that effective gun control measures result in little change in the volume of violence but a reduction in harm) would be too optimistic. The "hawks" would want us to believe that general restrictions on gun availability will increase both volume and harm from violence. But the hawks have not made a persuasive case.

The National Crime Victimization Survey (NCVS) is generally considered the most reliable source of information on predatory crime because it has been in the field continuously since 1973 and incorporates the best thinking of survey methodologists. From this source, it appears that use of guns in self-defense against criminal predation is rather rare, occurring on the order of 100,000 times per year.[22] Of particular interest is the likelihood that a gun will be used in self-defense against a home intruder. One study of data from the NCVS found that only 3% of victims were able to deploy a gun against someone who broke in (or attempted to do so) while they were at home.[23] Remembering that 40% of all households have a gun, we conclude that it is quite rare for victims to be able to deploy a gun against intruders even when they have one available.

Florida State criminologists Gary Kleck and Marc Gertz have offered a far-higher estimate of 2.5 million self-defense uses each year.[24] Indeed, Kleck and Gertz conclude that guns are used more commonly in self-defense than in crime. But Kleck and Gertz's estimate, and similarly large estimates from other surveys, may be too high. The problem stems from the fact that some misreporting is inevitable with any survey study, even of such mundane matters as the respondent's age, height, and weight or whether the respondent votes or uses a seat belt.[25] As Harvard professor David Hemenway notes, while surveys of defensive gun uses are likely to contain both "false negatives" (gun users who do not report their gun uses) and "false positives" (those who do not use a gun in self-defense within the recall period but report that they did),[26] the latter are likely to outweigh the former.[27] Suppose, for example, that one-half of one percent of all adults have actually used a gun in self-defense. In a survey of 5,000 adults, on average 25 people will have used a gun in self-defense and will have the chance to report a false negative, while the only misreporting option for the other 4,975 respondents is a false positive. If the false positive rate equals, say, 2% (which is credible in this case, given that some people will want to exaggerate their gun exploits to the interviewer), this survey will overstate the prevalence of defensive gun use by a factor of four even if *none* of those who have actually used a gun in self-defense report their uses.

An illustration of how even a low false-positive rate can lead to overestimates for rare events comes from a May 1994 survey of 1,500 adults conducted by ABC News and the *Washington Post*. In response to the question "Have you yourself ever seen anything that you believe was a spacecraft from another planet?" 10% of respondents answered in the affirmative. Around 1% of all respondents also indicated that they had themselves been "in contact with aliens from another planet,"[28] which is close to the proportion of respondents in Kleck and Gertz's survey who reported a defensive gun use.

There is direct evidence that surveys of defensive gun use also provide biased estimates. For example, the responses to a survey sponsored by the National Institute of Justice that used questions quite similar to those used by Kleck and Gertz seemed to imply that half of all rape attempts are foiled by a defensive gun use, and that the great majority of all potentially lethal assaults are stymied by gun-wielding victims.[29] The NCVS gives much lower estimates because it is designed to eliminate much of the possibility for false positives.[30]

If we believe that gun self-defense against assault is common, then it's reasonable to suggest that violent-crime rates, and the "success" rate in violent crime, may be reduced by the widespread possession of guns. We know from survey evidence that criminals do worry about the possibility of encountering an armed victim, and take care to avoid that possibility.[31]

Economist John Lott has led the way in promoting the claim that this deterrent effect, combined with the protective effect of self-defense, is so large as to support the conclusion in his book title *More Guns, Less Crime*.

Yet short of an outright ban on all firearms, most policy proposals preserve the right of adults without criminal records or histories of serious mental illness to keep guns at home for self-protection. Even a ban on handguns, the most dramatic policy change that receives mainstream support (by the *Washington Post* among others[32]) would still enable most people to keep long guns and shotguns at home to ward off intruders. More controversial are regulations that restrict the ability of private citizens to carry handguns away from home for self-protection or other reasons. While Lott and his coauthors claim that more gun carrying reduces violent crime, the best available evidence suggests otherwise.

Restrictions on Gun Carrying

Restrictions on gun carrying are prevalent and have a history that includes the famous requirement of the Wild West to "check your guns at the door" of taverns. In fact, the cowboys may have carried their guns while out on the prairie, but frontier towns introduced strict—and highly successful—gun-control measures to deal with rampant violence. Travelers were required by local ordinance to give up their guns before entering Dodge City and other cow towns.[33]

In modern times, there are a variety of restrictions on carrying guns into public places. A notable success in this regard, albeit one that has come at high cost, is the requirement that airline passengers pass through a metal detector before boarding. When this system was put in place, it stopped the epidemic of airline hijackings.

States and localities have gone further than restricting entry into public buildings; all but one state (Vermont) regulates the concealed carrying in any public place. Laws that delimit gun carrying together with police patrols to enforce these restrictions may reduce the number of fatal injuries by increasing the cost to criminals of carrying guns in public. These efforts may also save lives by reducing the chance that citizens who carry guns for self-protection wind up misusing the gun as part of an argument or fight.

Massachusetts' Bartley-Fox Amendment was an early effort to deter illicit carrying, and it has been subjected to several evaluations. The amendment took effect on April 1, 1975, and established a minimum sentence of one year for an initial violation of Massachusetts's legal requirements for carrying a gun away from home or office. The mandatory-sentence provision received tremendous publicity at the time it was implemented.

Glenn Pierce and William Bowers of Northeastern University assessed the impact of Bartley-Fox on violent crime through 1977.[34] They constructed annual time series on a number of violent-crime measures for Massachusetts, Boston, and several out-of-state comparison jurisdictions. They concluded that the short-term impact was to reduce the fractions of assaults and robberies involving guns and to reduce the criminal-homicide rate.

While police departments typically focus on keeping guns off the streets, in recent years over 30 states have enacted legislation that enables most citizens who are not prohibited from possessing a gun to obtain a concealed gun-carrying permit. Proponents of these laws argue that increasing the number of private citizens who carry concealed guns will deter crime, since criminals are not enthusiastic about the possibility of being shot by their victims, and note that relatively few people who have been issued concealed-carry permits misuse their guns. On the other hand, these laws may complicate law-enforcement efforts to prevent high-risk groups from carrying guns in public. These laws may also introduce an arms race between ordinary citizens and criminals. In their surveys of incarcerated felons, sociologists James Wright and Peter Rossi found that nearly two-thirds of those who used guns to commit their crimes reported that the prospect of encountering an armed victim was very or somewhat important in their decision to use a gun themselves.[35] Since guns are currently used in "only" around one-quarter of all robberies, 4% of sexual assaults and rapes, and 7% of assaults, permissive concealed-carry laws may have the negative consequence of increasing the proportion of criminals who use guns to commit their crimes.[36]

Whatever the effects of permissive concealed-carry laws on crime, they are likely to be small. Most of those who obtain concealed-carry permits are older, middle-income white males who live in rural areas[37]—a group that is already at relatively low risk for criminal victimization. Moreover, many of those who obtain concealed-carry permits already carried guns in public, so the actual change in the number of guns in public spaces may be modest. For example, survey data from North Carolina suggest that 85% of those with concealed-carry permits who carry a gun in their car and 34% of those who carry a gun on their person did so even before they obtained a permit, and most report that the frequency of gun carrying did not increase with the acquisition of a permit.[38]

The best available evidence suggests that permissive concealed-carry laws have little or no effect on violent crime and injuries.[39] In a widely publicized study, John Lott and David Mustard claim that permissive concealed-carry laws produce substantial reductions in violent crime.[40] Yet a reanalysis of their data by Dan Black of Syracuse University and Daniel Nagin of Carnegie Mellon shows that Lott and Mustard's statistical model confounds the effects of concealed-carry laws with the effects of other factors that are not adequately controlled for by Lott and Mustard's statistical models.[41] When Black and Nagin reanalyze Lott and Mustard's data using a more flexible statistical approach to control for these unmeasured factors, they find that the only statistically significant effect of permissive concealed-carry laws is an increase in criminal assaults.

Similar findings are obtained by Ludwig, who controls for unmeasured state-level variables by exploiting the fact that in every state only adults are eligible for concealed-carry permits.[42] As a result, any deterrent effects from permissive concealed-carry laws should be greater for adults than juveniles, and thus adult victimization rates should decline relative to what is observed for juveniles. Focusing on the *difference* between adult and juvenile victimization rates should be less susceptible to confounding factors, since unmeasured criminogenic variables should affect both adult and juvenile victimizations. The results suggest that permissive concealed-carry laws have a small, positive effect on adult homicide victimization rates, though this effect is not statistically significant.

So we return to our original conclusion, which can be summarized as, "Fewer Guns, Less Harm." The evidence to the contrary, no matter how often repeated and with what vehemence, does not stand up to close scrutiny. Our conclusion has direct implications for our analysis of the costs of gun violence. When we measure the benefits of interventions that reduce the prevalence of gun assaults, we assume that each gun assault is replaced by a knife attack (the most serious weapon that is typically substituted for guns in assaults). The savings to society come from the fact that knife assaults are about one-third as likely to result in the victim's death as those assaults that involve guns,[43] and on average have less serious consequences for survivors as well.

Suicide

While there is a substantial body of research suggesting that gun availability matters for the outcomes of assault, the evidence for suicide is more ambiguous. One difference is that suicides as a whole are probably less likely to be impulsive than assaults. While this may be less true for suicide attempts among teenagers, the evidence presented in Chapter 2 suggests that a substantial minority of those who attempt suicide do so in response to a serious health problem. These people may be determined to seek out equally lethal alternatives when guns are not readily available, alternatives such as hanging, drug overdoses, and jumping from tall buildings or bridges. These devices are more easily employed for use in suicide than assault.

Research has documented an association between suicide and gun ownership but has not provided a definitive demonstration that gun ownership is the *cause* of suicide. Arthur Kellermann and his associates demonstrated by use of a case-control study in three cities that those who commit suicides at home are more likely to have a gun than are their neighbors, and that this difference holds even after controlling for several other characteristics, such as drinking and drug use, that might help account for the suicide.[44] Garen Wintemute and his associates used California data to document a greatly elevated rate of gun suicide during the first few weeks after purchase of a handgun.[45] While this evidence is suggestive, the possibility remains of reverse causation (the gun is acquired with suicide in mind) or of some unmeasured "third cause" that links gun ownership and suicidal tendencies indirectly.

Given the lingering uncertainty about the effects of gun availability on suicide, we calculate our estimates for the costs of gun suicides using three different assumptions that should bracket the true costs. Our first set of estimates assume no weapon substitution—that is, when guns are somehow made unavailable for use in suicide, those who would have used a gun now give up the idea of suicide altogether. Our second set of estimates assume full replacement with equal harm—in this case, eliminating the use of guns in suicide has no net effect on the number of serious self-inflicted injuries, since people substitute toward mechanisms that are as lethal as guns. Our third set of estimates assume that those with serious health problems find some other equally effective way to inflict injuries on themselves, but the rest of the gun-suicide victims do not.

Summary for Weapon-Substitution Assumptions

Here, in sum, are our assumptions on weapon substitution and the consequences:

Assault: Allow for perfect weapon substitution. Since knives and clubs are less lethal than guns, the consequence is a large reduction in fatal injuries.

Unintentional: No substitution or replacement

Suicide: Ambiguous. We experiment with three different scenarios. Scenario 1: Allow for perfect weapon substitution for all suicide attempts, under the assumption that all suicides are premeditated. Assume that in each case the individual seeks out a method that is as lethal as firearms, so the result is no change in the number of fatal or nonfatal injuries. Scenario 2: Allow for no weapon substitution or replacement, under the assumption that all suicides are impulsive and that attempters are averse to nongun methods. The result is a full decrease in fatal and nonfatal suicides equal to the number of gun suicide attempts each year. Scenario 3: Allow for perfect weapon substitution for the estimated 40% of cases where the attempter may have a chronic illness. Assume no weapon substitution for the remaining cases.

If gun suicides on net have social costs to society, then scenario 1 for suicides will provide a lower-bound estimate for the costs of gun violence, scenario 2 is an upper-bound estimate, and scenario 3 is an intermediate estimate.

4

What Counts?

Gun-violence rates have declined sharply since 1993, and further reductions could surely be achieved if we were willing to make the necessary sacrifices. Just how much should government agencies expend in reducing gun violence? Tax revenues, regulatory authority, and law-enforcement resources all have other valuable uses. A systematic assessment requires that the benefits of reduced gun violence be translated into some metric that will allow comparison with the benefits of other uses of those resources. The most convenient metric is money.

Assigning a dollar value to the costs of gun violence turns out to be anything but routine. One problem is that much of the relevant losses from gun violence are not commodities traded in the marketplace, but rather personal losses such as pain, fear, and life itself. Analysts have used widely differing accounting principles and procedures in this and other contexts where life is at stake. In what follows, we develop an accounting framework that is comprehensive and consistent with the practices of cost-benefit analysis, even though it is quite different from the "Cost of Illness" framework that at one time represented the conventional wisdom in such matters.

The result is a method for assigning dollar values to a reduction in gun violence, or even to the total elimination of gun violence. Any reduction in the *costs* imposed by gun violence is, of course, a *benefit*, which can be compared with the magnitude of the investment required to achieve it.

Defining "Costs"

What do we mean when we talk about the "costs" of gun violence in America? A useful definition provides guidance for the specific problem that faces policymakers: What resources should be expended to combat gun violence? For example, suppose a county is considering the possibility of screening entrants to public buildings with a metal detector. The cost of metal detectors, attendants' wages, and inconvenience to the public must be weighed against the likely reduction in risk of gunshot injury to people who use the building. Our task, then, is to place a value on that change in risk.

Ideally we could measure the dollar value associated with a life-saving program by estimating the willingness to pay (WTP) for the program by all affected parties and then summing. In recent years, the WTP approach has been widely accepted by economists as the theoretically "correct" approach for cost estimates such as ours.[1] Consider two possible conditions, the *status quo* (A) and some alternative condition (B) that would result from a government program that reduces the prevalence of firearm injuries, such as the system for screening entrants to county buildings. The reductions in the prevalence of firearm injuries achieved by the program will affect both injury risks and standard of living. Some people will have lower injury risks with the program, as will their family members and friends, which makes them better off. Some people will also have lower tax bills or face lower prices because of the savings in shared medical expenses, the increased number of healthy survivors who are contributing to public goods and pension plans, and so forth. The aggregate WTP is the sum of what each individual in society would pay to achieve state B rather than A.[2] This conceptual approach must in practice be adapted to the limitations of available data.

All or Part

In some applications, it is useful to estimate the costs of *all* gun violence, rather than the costs associated with some part of the total that may be affected by a particular intervention. It is commonplace to hear estimates for the overall cost of other threats to the public health and safety. We are told that highway accidents in 1993 cost the American public $365 billion,[3] that the abuse of alcohol and drugs costs $246 billion in 1992,[4] that asthma is a $14 billion-per-year problem.[5] Such estimates may guide policymakers and the public about the relative burdens imposed by different afflictions. Knowing whether gunshot injuries are a $1 billion problem or a $100 billion problem overall is useful in making a "first cut" in setting public priorities and organizing a response.

Estimating the overall cost of gun violence entails imagining a condition in which there wasn't any. Specifying that alternative world requires information about the collateral changes produced by efforts to reduce gun violence, answers to questions like "Could guns be used to threaten others?" and "Would law enforcement officials be armed?" This is a fanciful exercise, though useful in clarifying some of the conceptual issues. The alternative approach is to analyze relatively small changes in gun violence that might be associated with a real intervention. Because we can observe actual interventions that produce small changes in gun violence, we can reasonably place a value on, say, a 1% reduction in gunshot injuries, and multiply that answer by 100 to provide a sense of the overall magnitude of the problem. But we don't expect that this second approach will necessarily give the same answer as attempting to estimate the overall costs directly, because the kinds of collateral changes associated with the complete elimination of gun violence may be quite different. In fact, estimating the overall costs directly is not even a well-defined question in the absence of a credible intervention that could accomplish the elimination of gun violence. Without defining such an intervention, we don't know what assumptions to adopt about other changes associated with the new regime.

Prevention and Avoidance

Of course, there have been instances where an important threat to the public health has been eliminated through concerted action by the government. Considering such an extreme change helps illuminate the full extent of the burdens that were imposed on society by the disease. For those of us from an older generation, the case that comes to mind most readily is polio.

Before an effective vaccine was developed, parents lived in fear that their children would be stricken with polio. By the time of the Great Depression, it was perhaps the most feared disease known. There was no cure, and it crippled or killed some of its victims. "All across America in the late 1940s and early 1950s, polio changed the face of childhood. Families fled the cities, swimming pools were closed, mothers fretted that an innocent frolic in a neighborhood creek could paralyze their child for life."[6] The polio epidemic peaked in 1952 with 58,000 new cases; between 1947 and 1959, 17,000 died and hundreds of thousands were disabled.

With the introduction of the Salk vaccine in 1955, and the more effective oral Sabine vaccine in 1961, polio was quickly eliminated. There has not been a naturally occurring case in the United States since 1979. The savings to society from this miracle include the costs avoided from acute and long-term medical care of victims, the suffering of victims and their families, and the lost productivity of those who died young or were permanently disabled. But the savings were not limited to the costs associated with suffering the disease—also important was the elimination of any need for families and public agencies to take precautions, or even to worry about the possibility of someone they cared about being stricken. In sum, the total cost to American society of living with polio, and the savings from eliminating polio, included both the consequences for actual victims, and the preventive measures taken by parents, schools, and other agencies when polio was a real threat.[7]

A more recent example illustrates the same point but, regrettably, in the opposite direction. AIDS emerged as a threat long after polio ceased to hold any sway over our anxieties.

Before the risk of HIV infection, sex could lead to all sorts of problems, but contracting a wasting, fatal disease was not one of them. That risk has now changed sex in this country. For example, in a nationally representative 1992 survey of American adults, 30% reported that they had changed their sexual behavior in response to the risk of AIDS; while the figure was somewhat higher for noncohabiting single adults, behavioral changes were reported even by around one in ten monogamous married couples.[8] We presume that the prevalence of these behavioral changes can only have increased during the last decade. Most remarkable has been the precautions that are now routine in preventing the remote chance of contagion through contact with tainted blood. In December 1991, the U.S. Occupational Safety and Health Administration (OSHA) issued a 178-page set of rules outlining precautions that employers must take to reduce the risk of infection in the workplace, motivated in part by the case of a woman in Florida who purportedly contracted the HIV virus from visiting her dentist.[9] The estimated costs of implementing these regulations, which include employer mandates to maintain medical records for "at risk" employees for up to 30 years following their separation from the firm are over \$800 million per year.

The analogy with gun violence is clear. While it is hard to imagine a "vaccine" that would erase gunshot wounds as a threat to the public health, let's consider the possibility as a thought experiment. The savings would include, as in the case of polio (and, potentially, of AIDS) both the elimination of costs stemming from victimization, and the elimination of any necessity of guarding against being shot or investing in gun-violence-prevention measures or even for worrying about the possibility of becoming a gunshot victim. Our point can be summarized as follows: *The total costs of the current volume of gun violence (as compared with a circumstance in which it had been eliminated) is equal to the costs stemming from gunshot woundings, plus the costs of all the efforts to deter shootings or protect against them.* Our shorthand for referring to these two categories will be "victimization costs" and "prevention costs." Thus

$$\textit{Total costs} = \textit{victimization costs} + \textit{prevention costs.}$$

As in the case of the Sabine vaccine, an intervention that somehow eliminated gun violence would have benefit equal to these total costs.[10]

In practice, we don't expect such miracles. Gun violence has always been a part of life in America, and the best we can hope for is to reduce, rather than eliminate, this threat. Even so, both types of costs remain relevant. Victimization costs will of course be reduced. And a reduction in the threat level will also reduce the need for prevention efforts. The savings will come in a reduced homicide caseload in the criminal-justice system, in a revival of violence-impacted neighborhoods, in the emotional relief to mothers now concerned about their children's safety. How the victimization and prevention costs tend to relate to the objective threat level is somewhat unclear. When there is no threat, those costs are zero—but do they increase in proportion to the threat from there? Some prevention activities have an all-or-nothing quality, such as moving to the suburbs or requiring that all building entrants pass through a magnetometer. And the psychology of risk also tends to introduce nonproportional effects in victimization: low-probability events tend to be either overweighted or ignored entirely.[11] As a result, it may be that there would be some disproportionate added benefit to the total elimination of gunshot violence, rather than reducing it to a fraction of its current level.

In what follows, we consider victimization and prevention costs in turn.

The Costs of Victimization

The traditional approach to estimating the social costs of illness (or, in our case, victimization) is to sum the "direct" costs (primarily medical treatment) and "indirect" costs. Indirect costs stem from the reduced productivity of victims, measured in the labor market by earnings. This approach has been called the "cost of illness" (COI) accounting framework, or sometimes the "human capital" method.[12] The COI approach has a long history, with the first COI study published as early as 1950, and over 200 such studies published by 1980.[13] It has been quite influential in public discussion about the costs of injuries in the United States, as evidenced by the prominent role played by COI in a 1989 report to Congress on the costs of injury.[14] But this approach has been widely criticized.

The most damning criticism is that the COI approach lacks a theoretical foundation that would relate it to any accepted definition of the public good.[15] Yet there is a guiding principle: in one interpretation, it is "implicitly based upon the maximization of society's present and future production.[16] An Institute of Medicine committee referred to this basic approach as "output accounting," noting the similarity to national product accounting methods.[17]

The problem is that in a liberal society we measure human welfare not by the sum of production, but rather by the sum of utility or well-being of members of society. The value of a person's life and health is not measured by productivity in the labor market, but must also take account of quality of life as judged by the individual.[18] The amount people are willing to sacrifice to reduce the risk of gun violence does not necessarily bear much relationship to their earnings.

Valuing Reductions in Injury Risk

Placing a monetary value on life is anathema to humanists who believe that it is priceless. But in everyday life, it's inescapably true that reducing threats to life and limb must contend with other goals. Scarce resources dictate a sort of "quality-quantity" tradeoff. In the public sector, for example, it is a routine matter to assign a value to life in making highway-design decisions, and information of this sort is increasingly taken into account in regulatory decision-making on environmental protection and other areas. In the private sector, product design is one arena where safety and economy may conflict. Occasionally a product-design decision will become public, as in the famous Ford Pinto case of the late 1970s. Ford Motor Company executives decided against recalling the Pinto for an $11 modification of the gas tank, guided by a study indicating that the costs of the recall would outweigh the benefits (burn deaths and injuries avoided) by $100 million. A jury that was informed of this study and its role in Ford's decision then awarded $125 million in punitive damages to a young man who had been badly burned by the explosion of such a gas tank. (The extra $25 million was interest.)[19] But just because the jury was repulsed by the cold-blooded accounting doesn't mean that the essential tradeoff can be denied.

Indeed, we all make implicit judgments about the value of our own lives and those of our family when we decide whether it's worth the extra money to buy additional safety features in motor vehicles, tools, bicycle helmets, and so forth. Should we buy the smoke detector that only signals fast flaming fires, or spend more to get one that also has a photoelectric capability to detect slow smoldering fires? And what about installing a carbon-monoxide detector while we're at it?

To be precise, such decisions entail a judgment, not about the value of a particular life, but rather the value of a small increase in the probability of death. Thomas Schelling begins his famous essay on this subject with the following distinctions: "It is not the worth of human life that I shall discuss, but of 'life-saving,' of preventing death. And it is not a particular death, but a statistical death."[20] If a million people are each willing to spend $5 on a device that will reduce the probability of death for each of them by one millionth (a "microrisk"), then the total of $5 million expended saves one life on the average; we conclude that a "statistical life" is worth that amount for this group of people. Five million dollars may be more than any one of them would or could pay to avoid certain death. But this "ransom" value of an *identified* life is not our concern: The public's willingness to pay for small increments of safety is what's relevant for valuing safety-enhancement programs. After all, when such programs are undertaken, no one knows which lives will be saved. Instead, the service provided by the safety program *ex ante* is that a large number of people enjoy a small reduction in risk.

A variety of techniques have been used to estimate how much people would be willing to pay for reducing the risk of injury or illness to themselves and their friends and relatives. We will consider four:

1. The *present value of future earnings* (or of consumption expenditures) is sometimes offered as a lower bound for the true value of life. The intuition rests on the belief that individuals would give up everything to avoid sure death; then assuming that the additional satisfaction derived from consumption (or "marginal utility") decreases as the standard of living increases, it is a simple exercise to show that a rational person, given the opportunity to buy a reduction of one percentage point in the chance of dying in the near future, would be willing to pay more than 1% of their lifetime consumption. The problem with this argument is that the premise is not correct; people would *not* pay everything to avoid a sure death. Below some consumption level, life is not worth living (or not possible). And that minimum consumption level at which we "break even on life" differs widely among individuals. For someone who is suicidal, their current consumption level is too little to sustain a wish to live, and they would pay nothing to avoid sure death. Others may be so in love with life itself that even the most meager subsistence level is viewed as preferable to death—and be willing to pay the entire difference between current income and subsistence to avoid sure death. Most of us are in between these two extremes.[21] In any event, the "lower bound" argument doesn't work as a justification for using an earnings measure.[22]

2. Another approach is to value lives saved from a particular intervention by using an estimate derived from the *analysis of relevant prices in the marketplace*. For example, a widely used approach is to examine the extra wage compensation that workers require in order to take risky jobs.[23] Other areas of study include prices of real estate[24] or consumer goods[25] as related to health risks. A review of the relevant literature places the value of one statistical life at between $3.75 and $8.75 million.[26]

These market-based studies can provide useful information about how people respond to risks if consumers and workers have accurate information about the health risks associated with different jobs, houses, and other consumer products. Economists assume that the market will provide an accurate indication of the public's tradeoff between safety and money; if the risk premium for a job were not sufficient given the preferences of the relevant group of workers, then the employer will have trouble recruiting an adequate supply of labor and, if too generous, would experience a surplus of applicants. Of course, if workers are generally misinformed about the risks of a particular job, then the risk premium will misrepresent those preferences.[27]

In practice it's a difficult statistical problem to partial out the effects of health risks on the wage structure from all the other influences. For example, jobs that have higher risks of death (for example, the construction of a new skyscraper) may have other features that will also affect the attractiveness of this work (such as exposure to the elements and hard physical labor), hence affecting the supply of labor and ultimately the wage for this occupation.[28] If any of the job attributes that affect wages and are correlated with health risks are unmeasured or poorly measured, analysts will mistakenly confound the wage effects of health risks with the effects of these other job characteristics. Similar problems can arise in studies that relate variation in health risks to the price of homes or other consumer goods.

Since there is little information available on how wages or other prices respond to the risks of gunshot injury,[29] the leading study on this subject inferred what people would pay for changes in these risks from generic studies of the value of life. Ted Miller and Mark Cohen estimated the cost of gunshot death based on estimates taken from other contexts.[30] There are several reasons to question the application of this approach to the case of gun violence. First, as we have seen, the victims of gun violence are not in any sense representative of the U.S. population. Those who commit suicide are indicating that they place no value on their lives (at least at the moment when they pull the trigger). Victims of gun assault often engage in such risky activity as to constitute probabilistic suicide—dealing drugs at an inner-city street corner is a form of Russian roulette.[31] And they tend to have poorer-than-average life prospects. In any event, values extracted from a study of the general population cannot be reliably applied to this population.

An alternative to using the average value for the general population of workers is to use values estimated from more comparable subpopulations. The adjustments could be of two forms. First, the observation that some gun-assault victims have chosen very risky occupations (drug dealing, for example) suggests that they place a relatively low value on their lives. Several studies have found that workers in high-risk occupations are a self-selected group who require relatively small compensation for those risks. On average the value they place on their lives is less than for workers who chose safer occupations. Such people are more likely than others to smoke or drive unbuckled, further evidence that they place a relatively low value on their lives.[32] If assault victims are more like workers in risky occupations than average workers, then by their own preferences a lower-than-average valuation is appropriate.

The second adjustment has to do with income. In general, and not surprisingly, those with lower incomes are willing to pay less than better-off individuals to avoid a small increase in the chance of injury. To the extent that gunshot victims tend to have low incomes, they will place a lower value on their own life than the average individual.

These adjustments are bound to be controversial. It can and has been argued that the government should use a uniform standard across population groups in regulating risk, without regard to income or preferences of the individuals involved. Risk regulation can then serve as a form of implicit income redistribution, giving the poor more safety than they would be willing to pay for (if given the choice of more safety vs. more of other things).[33]

3. Economists Ted Miller and Mark Cohen have pioneered the use of *jury awards to obtain estimates for the value of nonfatal gunshot wounds*. Using a sample of physical assaults that re-

sulted in a civil trial, Miller and Cohen estimate that each non-fatal gunshot injury imposes costs of around $170,000 on the victim, while the costs of nonfatal knife injuries are on the order of $70,000.[34]

There are several problems with such estimates. First, only a small proportion of personal-injury cases ever reach trial, and those that do are likely to be unrepresentative in various ways.[35] More importantly, the jury award is not a valid estimate of the social cost even in principle. The jury is being asked to answer a different question than the one facing policymakers. Cohen notes that the legal theory is "to give the injured party a sum of money which will restore him, as nearly as possible, to the position he would have been in if the wrong had not been committed; in other words, to make the plaintiff whole."[36] Cohen also notes that courts have recognized the problem that full compensation may be infinite in some cases, and have "refor-mulat[ed] the standard of compensation to be 'an amount such as a reasonable person would estimate to be fair compensation' and by allowing jurors wide latitude in determining the ulti-mate award. Moreover, instructions to juries apparently do not typically reflect the full compensation standard. Instead, jurors are given general instructions that permit them to award a 'fair' or 'reasonable' amount as compensation for pain and suffer-ing."[37] Thus, jury awards either overstate what people will pay to reduce the risks of injury (when juries are instructed to fol-low the full-compensation standard) or they bear no clear re-lation to the willingness-to-pay standard of public economics (when juries are given wide latitude to select a "fair" level of compensation).[38]

(4) Lastly, the method that we actually prefer for estimating the value of life and injury is to simply *ask people how much they are willing to pay for a reduction in the risk of gunshot injury.* We develop and implement this "contingent valuation" method in Chapter 8. While it, like the three methods discussed above, is somewhat controversial, it has the virtues of being directly relevant and relatively easy to interpret.

Concern about Others

The first three methods for valuing a reduction in gun violence (but not the fourth) share an artificial focus on the individual's concern about her own personal safety. But the public concern about gun violence has much to do with the safety of loved ones, neighbors, classmates, members of the same church or temple, public figures, and others who have enough of a personal connection that their death or injury would have emotional impact. Mutual concern enhances the value of creating a safer community.

The importance of these interpersonal concerns has the effect of further removing the valuation problem from objective to subjective judgment. A community that is closely interrelated by kinship, friendship, and other connections would place a higher value on eliminating a given threat than would an equally wealthy community of strangers. This point can be illustrated by a hypothetical example. Suppose a willingness-to-pay study was conducted in one of two ways with the 100 members of a college sorority. They are asked either:

A. How much are you willing to pay to avoid a one percent chance of your being shot tomorrow? Or
B. How much are you willing to pay to avoid one member of your sorority being selected at random and shot tomorrow?

While the two questions pose the same personal risk to each individual, the second broadens the field of concern and, we submit, would likely yield a higher WTP.[39] There is no double counting in this example—the value of the public good in question (greater safety) does depend on how much people care about each other, as well as how much they care about themselves.[40]

Sentiment is not the only reason why gunshot injuries may be a community problem. The injuries avoided from implementing a safety-enhancing program may affect the material standard of living as well as the level of safety in the community. To the extent that the safety-enhancing program affects net or "surplus" production, it has financial implications that go beyond the value of risk reduction per se. For a life saved or injury averted, the community gains whatever the individual produces over his remaining lifetime as well as the medical costs associated with that injury. But the community also "loses" the value of the individual's consumption of goods and services over his remaining lifetime. Whether on balance the "surplus" is positive or negative will depend on his circumstances and behavior.

In schematic form, we can define an individual's "Public Savings Rate" (PSR) as follows:

$$PSR = Production - Consumption$$

where *Production* is measured by earnings (gross of taxes) and *Consumption* is the sum of private consumption expenditures, all medical bills, and the value of other goods and services paid for by government and other third parties.

The basic question here is whether we have a tangible stake in the continued life and health of a stranger—whether that stranger, if she continues to live, will contribute more than she takes during her remaining years, in the sense of having a positive PSR. She might run a "deficit" by this standard because she is receiving nonwage income (pensions, income from investments) or spending down her net worth, or using more medical care than she pays for from insurance contributions and taxes.[41]

The intuition behind this measure is highlighted by considering the case of industrialist Andrew Carnegie. What would have been the financial costs to society had Carnegie been killed in a horse-and-buggy accident at the age of 15? The answer depends on what share of his earnings he would have spent on houses, yachts, trips, a fleet of Model T's, and other extravagances that have proven irresistible to the rich throughout the ages. If Carnegie would have consumed his entire fortune, then his premature death would arguably have had little effect on the material standard of living for everyone else. Yet as it turns out, Carnegie consumed far less than he produced. Since he wound up donating over 90% of his wealth to charitable causes,[42] a fatal accident at a young age would have noticeably reduced the quality of life for many others in the community.

To this calculation of net contribution to the community's assets we would want to add an accounting of contributions she would make outside of the marketplace. That would logically include both positive and negative contributions: raising kids and performing volunteer work (on the positive side) as well as criminal predation and unsafe driving (on the negative side). The monetary equivalents of such nonmarket "services" should be combined with the net financial consequence to get the bottom line.

While estimating the value of all such services seems like a daunting task, it may not be that important in practice. We explore this issue in some depth in Chapters 5 and 6, concluding that we don't have much of a tangible stake in the continued existence of strangers. Outside of altruistic concerns and concern about our own life chances, and those of friends and loved ones, it may make little difference to our quality of life if the death rate were reduced a bit across the board, except to increase the shared financial burden of supporting and caring for the elderly, financing the national debt and providing public goods such as national defense.[43] But if the change in death rate is not uniform—if, for example, those who tend to produce more than they consume are differentially affected—then the effect on the overall standard of living may be too large to ignore safely.

Still, we find that the greatest value of increased safety is not found in these sorts of calculations about net savings, but rather in our direct concern for our own personal safety and the safety of family and friends and perhaps others in the community. The value in this case is largely subjective. If we enjoy life, then we place value on anything that will increase the chance that we will go on living and avoid pain and disability. And the continued life and health of our family and friends is vital to our continued enjoyment. It may be unpleasant to contemplate placing a monetary value on this sentiment, but, as we have seen, it is implicit in day-to-day decisions that we do make.

Conclusions Regarding Victimization Costs

This discussion has identified problems with standard valuation methods and provided some guidance in developing a more reliable approach. For now, we note three lessons:

1. Victimization costs are best thought of in terms of the quality of life and health, as monetized, at least in principle, by the willingness of households to pay for reduced risk and its consequences.

2. Because communities are not autarkic collections of strangers, but rather linked through social and family connections, victimization costs include the concern individuals have for protecting the lives of others and not just themselves. And since households are connected through government tax and expenditure programs, insurance pools, the market for loanable funds, and nonmarket productive activity, community members may have a selfish stake in the health and well-being of strangers as well.

3. While in practice gunshot injuries are concentrated among certain groups defined by socioeconomic status, mental health, and criminal involvement, victimization costs do not necessarily follow those same contours. The costs of gun violence, properly understood, are prospective and subjective. A middle-aged mother living in the suburbs may place a higher value on reducing gun injuries than a 20-year-old drug dealer living in the inner city. While that reversal may seem strange at first, it is a natural consequence of a presumption that public value should be judged on the basis of private preferences.

The Costs of Prevention

Recall that the total costs of gun violence include not only the costs of actual victimization (however computed), but also the costs of preventing and defending against this type of violence. Should a "vaccine" be invented that eliminated the threat of gun violence, one major source of savings would be to eliminate any need for individuals, firms, or government agencies to adapt to this threat. Yet the value of these prevention costs have largely been ignored in previous studies of the costs of gun violence.

To illustrate the point, consider the costs of gun violence with respect to the president. In the "victim cost" sense, this cost has been zero; there have been no shootings since 1981, when President Reagan was wounded in the attack by John Hinkley. But during that time, the threat of gun violence has forced each of the presidents to limit the ways in which he engages with the public, and the Secret Service has spent many millions of dollars securing against assassination attempt when the president does choose to go out in public. Of course, this vigilance is not just a response to the threat of guns, but other weapons are less likely to pose a real threat—every president who has been wounded or killed in an assassination attempt was shot.

In the private sector, the costs are associated with reducing the individual risk of being shot. A number of decisions may be influenced by this threat, including residential and commercial location decisions, hours of operation for retail establishments, and family decisions about when and where to go out for the evening or to allow the children to play. In aggregate, the result may be blighted neighborhoods, playgrounds abandoned to gang members, business districts that close down at sunset, reduced tax collections for cities, and other all-too-familiar woes of urban life.

A nation with less gun violence would be different in many ways. Miami would have more international tourists, public schools would have an easier time recruiting teachers, taxi drivers might be more willing to take passengers to inner-city neighborhoods. While such problems are by no means caused by gun violence alone, gun violence exacerbates trends that would result in a world where crime was perpetrated solely with knives and other weapons, and thus less lethal than what is currently observed in the United States.

We return to the problem of estimating prevention and victimization costs in Chapters 7 and 8, respectively. First, however, we focus on the tangible victimization costs that have dominated the previous public health literature—medical expenses and lost productivity. We demonstrate that these tangible costs are far smaller than previous studies would suggest, which also suggests that surplus production is a proportionately small part of the overall problem.

5

Medical Costs

Gross versus Net

By design, firearms can inflict terrible damage on the human body. While the majority of all gunshot injuries are not fatal, survivors frequently face the prospect of a lengthy recovery period and even permanent disability. Two recent victims admitted to Grady Memorial Hospital in Atlanta are typical of the more serious cases. One was a 39-year-old male who was shot repeatedly as part of an argument. He was admitted to the hospital at 2:45 A.M. with wounds to the hip, thigh, abdominal wall, thorax, diaphragm, and liver. Doctors cleared his chest cavity of blood, reinflated his lung (which had been collapsed by one of the bullet wounds), and cleared out substantial amounts of damaged (and no longer viable) tissue from his liver, diaphragm, and abdomen. His initial treatment and recovery required a 13-day hospital stay, at which time he was discharged and returned home. Complications led to a rehospitalization of an additional seven days, as well as 11 doctor's office visits during the first year following his injury.

While the first victim eventually experienced nearly a full recovery, the victim in our second example, a 27-year-old male was not so lucky. He was shot several times in the neck as part of a criminal assault, resulting in spinal cord damage. After five days in the hospital's intensive care unit and another ten days in an acute-care ward, he was discharged to a spinal-cord rehabilitation center, where he spent the next 90 days. He is now a quadriplegic.

Needless to say, medical treatment for such cases is costly; the lifetime costs for the second case may easily exceed $1 million. The constant flow of gunshot injuries impose a considerable burden on the trauma centers in large cities, and hence on the taxpayers, since almost all such patients are medically indigent. In seeking to come to grips with the social costs of gun violence, the burden on the medical-care system seems like a good place to begin.

Yet in the larger scheme of things, the additional medical costs do not deserve much prominence in the argument for taking gun violence seriously. Here we document a total-cost estimate of about $2 billion per year, surely not trivial, yet not of great significance compared to either the nation's total medical bill (more than $1 trillion) or, more importantly, compared with the value of lost life and peace of mind. Further, the *net* cost of gunshot wounds to the medical-care system is substantially less than $2 billion, as explained below.

Gross Costs of Medical Treatment

Compiling estimates for the costs of treating gunshot wounds requires a variety of data sets and a number of assumptions. The result is necessarily imperfect, but our calculations, first published in the *Journal of the American Medical Association* in a paper coauthored with Bruce Lawrence and Ted Miller,[1] improve on previous estimates for the costs of treating gunshot injuries in several ways. We use the most up-to-date and comprehensive data sources available, including some that have not been used for this purpose before. One challenge in developing good estimates is that the distribution of costs is highly skewed, with a relatively few million-dollar cases accounting for a large share of the total; a separate data source on spinal-cord injuries provided detail on these catastrophic cases. Another challenge is in distinguishing between medical *costs* and medical *charges* or payments; the latter may be quite different due to the cross-subsidy schemes employed by hospitals and other medical providers. We are able to use cost data for the most part.

The goal here is to estimate the annual *incidence* of medical costs resulting from gunshot injuries. Since spinal-cord and other permanent injuries generate a stream of extra medical costs stretching decades into the future, it is necessary to specify an accounting rule for aggregating expenses over time. We converted lifetime costs into a present value using a 3% "real" annual discount rate (abstracting from inflation), in accordance with the recommendation of the Panel on Cost-Effectiveness in Health and Medicine convened by the U.S. Public Health Service in 1993.[2]

All estimates are adjusted for inflation in the prices of medical goods and services through 1998 using the Consumer Price Index for Medical Care. The specific details of our estimation procedure, which draws on a number of local and national data sources, are presented in Appendix B.

Figure 5.1 presents the average medical costs for each of the three categories of injuries—gun assaults, suicides, and unintentional shootings—and for all gunshot wounds. These calculations include the full lifetime medical costs of treating patients, from emergency transport to emergency department and hospital costs through long-term follow-up care. The pattern of average costs across the three categories reflects the differing case-fatality rates because fatal injuries are less costly than nonfatal injuries. Self-inflicted gunshot injuries, with their high case-fatality rate, average $5,400, while gun-assault injuries average $18,400, and unintentional shootings $22,400.

Figure 5.2 depicts the total lifetime medical costs of treating gunshot injuries. The 113,000 gunshot wounds that were incurred in 1997 will ultimately generate $1.9 billion in treatment costs over the course of the victims' lives. As shown in this figure, the medical costs of treating gunshot injuries are driven largely by nonfatal injuries (64,000 out of 113,000 of which are assaults). Remarkably, fully 60% of the total costs of treating gunshot victims are accounted for by the 2% of all gunshot wounds that involve injury to the spinal cord.

While gunshot injuries themselves are concentrated largely among the young and those with low incomes (chapter 2), the costs of providing medical treatment for victims is shared widely. Figure 5.3 shows that around half of the costs of treating gunshot wounds is borne by government programs, and thus

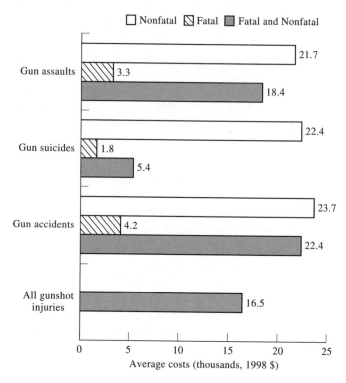

Figure 5.1. Average Medical Treatment Costs per Gunshot Injury ($thousands). Data from various state and national sources (see Appendix Table B1).

passed on to the public in the form of higher taxes. Another fifth is borne by private health insurance programs and hence passed along to policyholders in the form of higher premiums.

Net Medical Costs

The estimates reported above provide an answer to the question "What are the total annual costs of treating gunshot victims?" That is not the same as asking what effect gunshot injuries have on the nation's total annual medical bill. This is because the

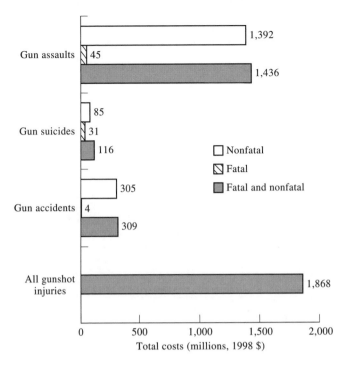

Figure 5.2. Total Medical Treatment Costs for Gunshot Injuries, 1997 ($millions). Data from various state and national sources (see Appendix Table B1).

savings to the medical system from eliminating gun violence equal the lifetime medical costs incurred by gunshot victims, less the medical costs that victims *would have* experienced had they *not* been shot. In what follows, we develop an estimate for this net effect of gun violence on aggregate medical spending and then conclude by discussing the question that is most relevant to our task—what financial burden do these medical costs impose on other members of the community?

The Net Effect on the Nation's Medical System

The net effect of gun violence on the nation's trillion-dollar medical bill requires some assumptions about what medical

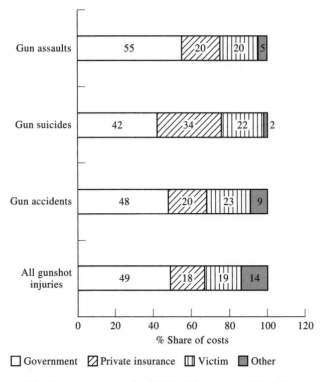

Figure 5.3. Payment Sources for Medical Treatment of Gunshot Wounds. Data from various state and national sources (see Appendix Table B1).

spending would be under the counterfactual scenario in which gun misuse is eliminated. Following our practice (Chapter 4), we assume that gunshot wounds from assault would be replaced one-for-one by wounds inflicted with other weapons and that gun suicides would follow one of three replacement paths, while there would be no substitution for unintentional shootings.

We also assume that those people who escape injury altogether once gun misuse has been eliminated have the same average life expectancy as other people in the general population of the same sex, age, race, and educational attainment, and that annual medical expenses would be equivalent to what we observe for men and women in the general population.[3] Under these assumptions, the present value of lifetime medical expenses (accounting for the victim's sex and age) is about $33,592 for gun homicide victims, $33,233 for unintentional shootings, and $35,612 for suicides. In reality, people at high risk for gunshot injury probably have below-average life expectancy, above-average risk for other costly injuries and illnesses, and limited health insurance coverage.[4] There is insufficient information to judge whether the net bias caused by these different sources of error is positive or negative.[5]

Also relevant is what happens when gunshot injuries claim the lives of workers, because those who replace the victim in his job may add to society's aggregate medical bill. When a Chicago construction worker is shot in a barroom fight, presumably his position will eventually be filled by someone else— either a Chicago resident or through immigration into the Chicago area. This "replacement" scenario is more dubious in the case of the national economy, but the fact is that immigration, both legal and illegal, represents a large source of human capital that is to some extent sensitive to the conditions of the labor market. It would be quite reasonable to assume that workers lost to gun violence can be readily replaced from the international pool. The bottom line is that in cases where fatally injured victims are replaced in their jobs by new entrants into the community, there is no "savings" to society from the reduction in medical services that the victim would have consumed had he not been shot because this medical spending is now redirected toward the replacement worker.[6]

On the other hand, if fatally injured workers are replaced by unemployed members of the local economy (who would have imposed costs on the local medical care system in any event), then the net effects of the gunshot wound on the medical system are similar to those associated with a fatal injury to someone who is not working—equal to the costs of treating the injury, less the lifetime medical costs that the victim would have incurred had he not been shot.[7] Since we have no way of knowing how fatally injured workers will be replaced, we develop all of our estimates under the two extremes that define the possible continuum—full replacement through immigration and full replacement from the local unemployment rolls. (See Appendix B for additional details.)

With these assumptions in hand, Figure 5.4 presents our estimates for the net costs to the medical system from gun assaults, suicides, unintentional shootings, and all gunshot injuries. Our "upper-bound" estimates for net medical costs come from assuming that every worker who is killed by gunfire is replaced through immigration and that there will be perfect weapon substitution for suicides when guns are made unavailable for misuse. The "lower-bound" estimates for net costs as-

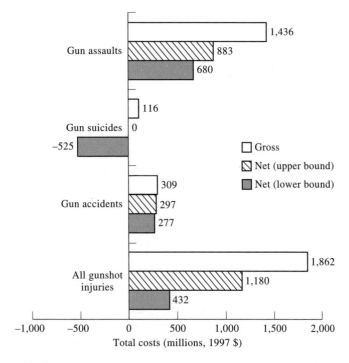

Figure 5.4. Gross vs. Net Medical Costs of Gun Violence, 1997. Data from various state and national sources (see Appendix Tables B1 and B5).

sume injured workers are replaced by unemployed residents of the local area and that there is no weapon substitution for suicides.

As seen in Figure 5.4, the net medical costs of the 77,923 assault-related gunshot injuries in the United States in 1997 range from $680 to $883 million—equal to 47 and 61% respectively, of the gross costs of treating gun-assault victims for their injuries.

The difference between net and gross medical costs is even more striking in the case of gun suicides, with net costs that range from $0 to $525 million. (That is, the second figure implies that the elimination of gun violence would actually increase aggregate medical spending in the United States by $525 million.) Gun suicides may reduce total medical spending because most victims of fatal gun suicides would have consumed far more in medical services during the remainder of their lifetimes had they not inflicted on themselves these injuries. This grim accounting does *not* mean that gun suicides make society "better off"—such a judgment would require a value system that emphasized the minimization of medical spending over all other considerations. In fact, our finding that gun suicides may "save money" for the medical system is in itself evidence that medical costs are a poor measure of the real burden that gun violence imposes on society.

The Net Effect on the Shared Financial Burden

Why has medical spending commanded such attention in public discussions of the cost of gun violence? As we argued in Chapter 4, medical expenses are usually a minor issue to those who are shot, compared with the pain, suffering, disability and emotional costs associated with gunshot injuries. The salience of medical costs in the public debate stems from the knowledge that they are paid by "third parties"—the rest of us. Using the concept introduced in Chapter 4, the victim's *Public Savings Rate* is generally reduced by the amount of the injury-related medical costs.

But the concern that the medical costs from gunshot injuries are a financial burden on the rest of the community is to an extent misplaced. Once again we need to consider the net effect rather than the gross effect, taking account of the counterfactual: if the victim had *not* been shot, then what would his lifetime medical costs have been, minus the payments he would have made to finance those medical costs (including self-pay amounts, medical insurance premiums, and payroll taxes). Because we subtract off these hypothetical payments, we can be assured that the effect of gunshot medical costs on the shared financial burden is less than the effect on the nation's total medical bill.

A numerical example may help illustrate the point. Suppose a 25-year-old construction worker is shot and dies after a week in the hospital, incurring medical costs of $10,000 paid for by insurance. If he had not been shot, his subsequent lifetime medical expenses would have been $30,000, of which he would have paid $20,000. For now, we ignore the possibility of immigration and calculate three measures of medical cost:

(1) $10,000   Cost of treatment for the gunshot wound

(2) −$20,000 Net effect on the nation's medical bill

(3) $0   Net effect on the shared burden of medical cost

The second measure nets the savings stemming from the man's death ($30,000 in lifetime costs) against the cost of treating the wound. The third measure takes account of the contribution he would have made to these lifetime medical expenses ($20,000), which is of course lost due to his death.

If the wound were *not fatal* and he recovers fully after incurring $10,000 in medical cost, and pays off $2,000 of his own medical bills, then the three measures are:

(1) $10,000 Cost of treatment

(2) $10,000 Net effect on the nation's medical bill

(3) $8,000   Effect on the shared burden

Returning to the first scenario where the victim dies, we can modify the example to allow for the possibility that his job will be filled by someone else. If it is filled by a foreign immigrant with the same profile of future medical expenses and payments, then the cost is $10,000 by any definition.

The difference between the second and third measures stems from the possibility that the decedent would have contributed something to paying future medical expenses had he lived. That payment is of no consequence in calculating the net effect on the nation's total medical expenditures, but does matter in accounting for the shared burden (except in the case of replacement by a foreign immigrant). So the shared burden is somewhat larger than the net effect on the nation's medical bill, but probably less than the gross cost of treatment for the gunshot injury (since gunshot victims as a group are unlikely to be paying their way on even routine medical expenses).

We make no further attempt here to estimate the shared burden. It is less than $2 billion—probably substantially less—and hence we can safely conclude that medical care accounts for only a small portion of the costs of gun violence.

6

The Mythical Importance of Productivity Losses

The labor market provides most adults with opportunities to engage in productive activity, at a wage reflecting their ability, experience, physical strength, character, and other attributes. A healthy 20-year-old may look forward to four or five decades in the labor market. The present value of this stream of earnings can be interpreted as the value of her "human capital," an asset in some ways comparable to a machine or other physical capital. The value of this human capital may be lost because of death or severe disability.

Gunfire injures or kills thousands every year and, barring compensatory immigration, shrinks the labor force accordingly. The loss of productive capacity has traditionally been counted as the predominant economic cost of illnesses and injuries that affect those of working age. While we (like other economists) reject this "cost-of-illness" accounting framework, favoring instead the willing-to-pay approach, we acknowledge that numbers on lost earnings are a common input in the public-policy process.

Furthermore, earnings do in fact play a role in the accounting framework we develop in chapter 4, though only in the context of the Public Savings Rate (PSR), defined as the difference between "production" and "consumption." In the discussion below, we first develop "human capital" estimates and then turn to the PSR calculation.

Earnings Losses from Gun Violence

Under the cost-of-illness framework, "an individual is seen as producing over time a stream of output valued at market earnings or by the imputed worth of housekeeping services. The human capital concept assumes a social perspective . . . [and] is useful for answering questions regarding the economic burden of a disease for a specific time period . . . or for determining the savings of a specific procedure or intervention program that will reduce illness and/or improve survival rates."[1]

Published estimates have incorporated the assumption that gunshot victims would have had the same earnings as other Americans of the same sex and age.[2] The motivation for this set of assumptions is pragmatic: for years, the only sociodemographic information available about gunshot victims was sex, age, and perhaps race from the Vital Statistics census of deaths. Yet as we show in what follows, this assumption results in substantial overestimates of lost market earnings for gunshot victims.

We begin by reexamining the losses in labor market productivity from fatal gunshot injuries. The 1993 National Mortality Followback Survey (NMFS) dataset discussed in Appendix A provides information on earnings prospects and sociodemographic characteristics of victims. Information about the American population as a whole comes from the 1993 Current Population Survey (CPS), March Demographic File, which provides detailed sociodemographic details about a random sample of 254,000 people.

It should be noted that the implicit assumption behind this general approach is that earnings reflect the social value of an individual's productivity. A vast literature in economics is devoted to exploring the theoretical and empirical basis for this assumption. Suffice it to say that the association between earnings and productivity is approximate at best, as most people can attest from personal observation in their own place of work. Of particular concern is the possibility that the labor market systematically undervalues entire groups, such as women, racial minorities, those with criminal records, and so forth. But while earnings is far from a perfect measure of productivity, the evidence does not point to large biases.[3]

As we see in Figures 6.1 through 6.3, gunshot victims are quite different from other people with respect to several sociodemographic characteristics that are correlated with earnings—employment during the previous year, marital status, and educational attainment. The figures are for males ages 18–29; the patterns for older men and for women are similar (see Appendix C).[4] Gunshot victims have lower earnings potential than members of the general population with respect to these measures. For example, Figure 6.1 shows that male gun-homicide victims ages 18 to 29 are half as likely as other men of the same age to be married (12 versus 24%), more than twice as likely to have dropped out of high school (44 versus 20%), and less likely to have worked during the last year (51 versus 72%). Figures 6.2 and 6.3 tell a similar story for the victims of unintentional fatal firearm injuries and for firearm-suicide victims.

Figure 6.4 presents estimates for the value of lost earnings and household production[5] for fatal gunshot injuries. When we assume that gunshot victims would have had the same lifetime earnings as people in the general population of the same sex and age,[6] estimated losses equal $810,000 for men and $520,000 for women. But when the analysis is refined to take account of race and educational attainment, then the estimated earnings and household-production losses from fatal gunshot injuries drop to around $580,000 and $460,000.[7]

The estimates presented above may still overstate the productivity that gunshot victims would have had if they were not shot, since victims have lower earnings during the year before death than other people of the same sex, age, race, and schooling. One possibility is that whatever factors are responsible for these earnings differences prior to death would persist throughout the course of the victim's life had he not been shot. This adjustment would imply losses of around $490,000 and $380,000 for male and female victims, respectively (Figure 6.4). Alternatively, gunshot victims may have lower earnings than other people during the year before their deaths for reasons that

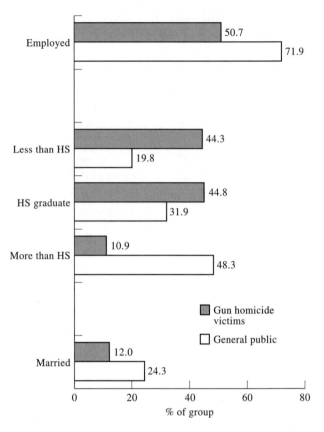

Figure 6.1. SES Characteristics of Gun Homicide Victims and the General Public: Males, 18-29. Data provided by the Vital Statistics and the National Mortality Followback Survey, National Center for Health Statistics, and the Current Population Survey.

are transitory. If the earnings of victims would have converged to those of others with similar characteristics had they not been shot, then the somewhat higher estimates presented above ($580,000 and $460,000) are more appropriate. Yet in either case, our calculations suggest that previous studies that ignore important sociodemographic differences between gunshot victims and other people will overstate the earnings and household production lost to gun violence.

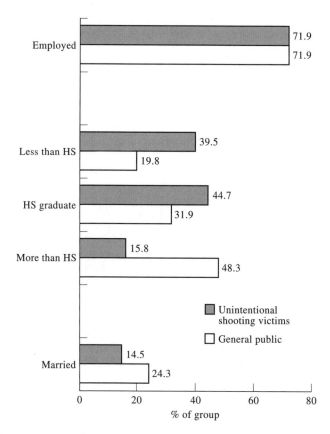

Figure 6.2. SES Characteristics of Unintentional Shooting Victims and the General Public: Males, 18-29. Data provided by the Vital Statistics and the National Mortality Followback Survey, National Center for Health Statistics, and the Current Population Survey.

The total productivity loss associated with gunshot wounds in 1997 is computed in Appendix C. Estimating lost earnings based on sex and age of the victims, the total loss is $26.6 billion. If we also take into account ethnicity and education, the total loss is just $19.5 billion. If workers tend to be replaced by immigrants on a one for one basis, then the loss in national product drops to approximately nil. For example, a large share of all working-age males were killed by gunfire in Germany

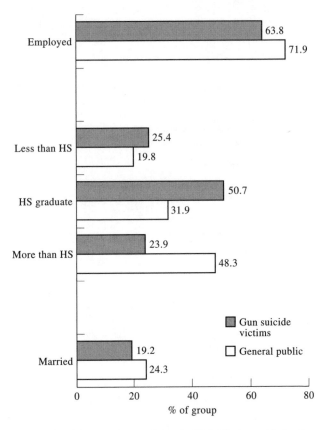

Figure 6.3. SES Characteristics of Gun Suicide Victims and the General Public: Males, 18-29. Data provided by the Vital Statistics and the National Mortality Followback Survey, National Center for Health Statistics, and the Current Population Survey.

during World War II. Germany nonetheless managed to rebuild its economy and become one of the most affluent nations in Europe, thanks in large part to immigration from Turkey and other countries. Yet the fact that the long-term consequences of the war on Germany's national output may have been surprisingly modest does not imply that the conflict did not impose dramatic costs on the populace. This result helps demonstrate that the cost-of-illness approach is based on a profound mis-

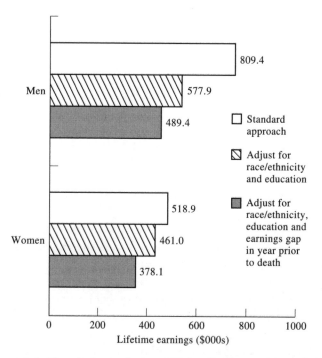

Figure 6.4. Three Estimates for Lost Lifetime Earnings and Household Production, Victims of Fatal Gun Injuries: Men and Women. Data provided by the Vital Statistics and the National Mortality Followback Survey, National Center for Health Statistics, and the Current Population Survey.

understanding of the real costs of injuries and illness to a society.

Netting Out Consumption

The larger concerns with the cost-of-illness approach are conceptual rather than data-related. In Chapter 4, we conclude that the financial effect of a death on the larger community is defined by the Public Savings Rate concept. It is the present value of future "Public Savings" that constitutes the burden on others' standard of living. That "burden" may be positive or negative, depending on whether the individual contributes more in production than he takes.

We began to implement that standard in the previous chapter's discussion of medical costs. The stakes are far higher in the case of productivity.[8] Focusing on net consumption has the effect of substantially reducing cost-of-illness estimates, since the U.S. personal savings rate is negligible—on the order of 5 or 6% in recent years (consisting primarily of retirement contributions),[9] and presumably even lower among gunshot victims, who as a group have below-average lifetime earnings.

In principle, we need also account for nonmarket production. The usual approach focuses on labor-market earnings, and accounts for only one form of production that is not generally traded in the marketplace—household production. Yet had they not been shot, gunshot victims would have engaged in a number of other productive activities that occur outside of the market. Many victims would have provided valuable services to society by raising children, caring for aging parents, or providing assistance to their neighbors. Other victims would have coached Little League, worked in a soup kitchen or donated their time to some other volunteer organization, as do 48.8% of all Americans for 4.2 hours per week on average.[10] Unfortunately, not all of the production that is lost to gun violence need be productive. Studies of gun homicide victims suggest that a majority have prior criminal records. Presumably some of these victims would have continued to participate in crime had they not been shot,[11] leading to a type of "negative production" that in principle should be taken into account, as should other destructive behaviors.

The bottom line, then, is that the loss of productivity resulting from gun injuries has in the aggregate little or no effect on the standard of living of others in the community. This conclusion follows from the assumption that the victims on the average were consuming as much as they produced. It is reinforced if we admit the possibility of worker replacement through immigration.

Where productivity and earnings *are* important is in financing an individual's actual and potential expenditure on reducing the risks of gun violence. The value of reducing injuries resides primarily in this subjective valuation, which may be correlated with earnings but leads to quite different conclusions in the aggregate, as we shall see.

7

Avoidance and Prevention

The most obvious costs of gun violence are those related to the tangible consequences experienced by victims—medical costs and lost earnings. Yet these are only a small part of the overall problem, as we demonstrated in the previous two chapters. The *threat* of gun violence imposes costs on all Americans, even those who are not actually victimized, because most people and many government agencies engage in costly behaviors designed to reduce the risk of gunshot injury. In what follows, we discuss some of the ways in which the preventative behaviors made by private citizens and public institutions reduce the overall quality of life in the United States. While we cannot quantify all (or even most) of these costs, our review suggests that they may be substantial.

Government Prevention Costs

Arguably the most fundamental job of government is to enforce the rule of law, which is accomplished largely by deterring misbehavior through the punishment of criminal transgressions. One important feature of the criminal justice system in the United States and most other developed countries is that more serious crimes are punished more heavily than less serious crimes, to create disincentives for criminals to increase the severity of their crimes. For example, if both robbery and murder were capital offenses, the extra (or marginal) cost to robbers of killing their victims—who are potential eyewitnesses—would be zero. Because murders are more costly to investigate, prosecute, and punish than robberies and assaults, and since guns intensify criminal attacks, gun violence increases the costs of administering the criminal justice system in the United States. We estimate this additional cost to be over $2 billion per year. Government agencies also engage in more obvious preventive activities by, for example, providing law enforcement officers with bulletproof vests. Expenditures of this type cost taxpayers at least another $1 billion per annum.

The Criminal Justice System and Deterrence[1]

Guns increase the costs of administering the criminal justice system in America by increasing the likelihood that criminal assaults result in the death of the victim.[2] Table 7.1 shows that the average incarceration costs per homicide ($244,000) far exceeds the figure for those aggravated assaults that are serious enough to be made known to the police ($6,200). These cost differences arise because people are far more likely to be arrested, tried, convicted, and sentenced to prison when they commit homicides rather than aggravated assaults.[3] Our calculations understate the difference in criminal justice costs between homicides and aggravated assaults because the former will also have higher investigation, pretrial, and trial costs, and the costs per year incarcerated may be higher for convicted murderers since they are likely to be assigned to higher-security (and thus more costly) facilities.[4]

These estimates suggest that eliminating the use of guns in crime will reduce criminal justice costs by at least $31,000 for every gunshot injury that is prevented. To see how we arrive at this figure, consider the effects of some intervention that results in 100 fewer gunshot injuries. Previous studies suggest that on average, every 100 assault-related gunshot injuries will result in around 20 deaths. To be conservative, we assume that every one of the 100 gunshot injuries that are prevented are replaced by 100 nongun injuries, of which around seven on

Table 7.1

Criminal Justice Costs of Homicide vs. Aggravated Assaults for 1996

	Homicide	Aggravated assault
Number of crimes known to the police	19,645	1,029,814
Number of people convicted & sentenced to prison/jail	11,178	50,262
Number of people incarcerated per crime	0.57	0.05
Average prison term (years)	10.7	3.1
Average cost per year in prison	$40,000	$40,000
Incarceration costs per crime known to the police	$243,960	$6,200

Notes: Estimates for the number of crimes known to the police from FBI (1997). Estimates for the number of people sentenced to prison/jail and the average time expected to be served from Brown (1999). Estimates for the average cost per year in prison from Donohue and Siegelman (1999); our calculation is likely to understate the difference in incarceration costs, since convicted murderers will probably be assigned to higher-security (and thus more costly) prisons and jails than those convicted of aggravated assault. Incarceration costs per crime known to the police thus equal $(0.57) \times (10.7) \times (\$40,000) = \$243,960$ for murder and $(0.05) \times (3.1) \times (\$40,000) = \$6,200$ for aggravated assault.

average will be fatal.[5] The savings to the criminal justice system from eliminating 100 gunshot injuries thus equal the difference between the criminal justice costs of 13 homicide cases ($3.2 million) and the costs of 13 nonfatal aggravated assaults ($80,600). Our estimated figure per gunshot injury comes from dividing this figure (around $3.1 million) by 100.

To put this figure into perspective, in Chapter 5 we estimated that the net effect of assault-related gunshot injuries on medical expenditures in the United States is somewhere between $9,000 and $11,000 per injury.[6] Thus, for each gunshot injury that can be prevented, the savings from reductions in criminal justice costs are around three times the savings in medical spending. Eliminating all gun violence in the United States as a whole in 1997 would have reduced the costs of administering the criminal justice system by at least $2.4 billion.

Security and Prevention

Most government agencies are charged with the job of protecting their employees, and some are further responsible for the safety of the public at large. Some portion of the expenditures made by these government organizations would be reduced or eliminated altogether in a world without gun violence. Quantifying these potential savings is difficult either because government agencies do not collect data on their current level of preventative expenditures or because it's not clear how these expenditures would change in response to a reduction in gunshot injuries. Instead, in what follows we provide readers with a rough sense of the potential magnitude of these savings by reviewing the types of expenditures that government agencies make in response to the threat of gun violence.

Schools Many children in the United States, particularly poor children in high-crime urban areas, are required to walk through metal detectors on the way into school each day. While this practice may enhance the safety of children, it may also affect the morale of students and teachers and detract from the educational climate of the school. Metal detectors may also directly affect student learning by taking away from class time, since security precautions increase the complexity of moving students in and out of classroom buildings,[7] and draw resources away from other instructional-related items such as the hiring of additional teachers or new textbooks.

Consider, for example, the security expenditures made by the Chicago public school system. Each of the city's 69 public high schools has a walk-through metal detector that cost between $2,500 and $3,000 to purchase. The Chicago public school system also employs 994 full-time security personnel who each cost the system around $25,000 per year,[8] in addition to 445 off-duty Chicago police officers who work part-time for the schools at an annual cost of around $15,500[9] and 140 full-time police officers from the Chicago Police Department's Youth Division who are permanently assigned to the public schools at an annual cost of around $67,000.[10] The Chicago public school system thus spends around $41 million each year for school security personnel, in addition to the costs of purchasing and maintaining metal detectors. While some of these preventive measures would stay in place even if gun misuse was eliminated, since knives and box-cutters will still pose a threat to student safety, the level of expenditures would almost surely be lower in a world without gun violence.

Law Enforcement In Washington, D.C., every officer in the Metropolitan Police Department is checked before they go out on patrol to ensure that they are wearing a bulletproof vest. While these vests may have secondary benefits in protecting officers against attacks with knives and other weapons, they are worn primarily for protection against gunshot injuries. Bulletproof vests typically cost between $400 and $700 each[11] and, if the practice of the D.C. police department is any guide, are used for around five years before they are replaced. If other police departments follow similar practices, then law enforcement in the United States as a whole may spend as much as $100 million each year to provide police officers with bulletproof vests (Table 7.2).[12]

Law enforcement agencies are also charged with the job of protecting high-level government officials. It seems reasonable to believe that the job of the Secret Service to protect the pres-

Table 7.2
Government Preventative Expenditures for Gun Violence

Security precaution	Expenditures
Airport security[a]	$720 million
Secret Service	FY 99 $613 million
ATF	FY 99 $558 million
Kevlar vests for law enforcement (annual expenditures for replacement of vests)	$100 million

Notes:
[a] In 1998 dollars. Figure accounts for metal detectors, X-ray machines and personnel, taken from Laband and Sophocleus (1992).

ident would be somewhat easier (and less costly) if gun violence were no longer a threat. Unfortunately, we have no way of determining exactly how much of the Secret Service's approximately $600 million annual budget (Table 7.2) is devoted to protecting public officials, or how much lower these expenditures would be if gunshot injuries were eliminated. But in any case Secret Service expenditures may be the least of the costs incurred with protection of the president; for example, every time the president ventures out in public, traffic patterns must be rearranged (a particularly severe problem with presidential visits to Manhattan), local law-enforcement support is required, and other members of the public are subject to metal detection, background checks, and other security precautions.

A slightly less glamorous government function is the enforcement of federal gun regulations. These regulations are enforced by the Bureau of Alcohol, Tobacco, and Firearms (ATF), an agency with an annual budget of around $550 million (Table 7.2). While we cannot determine the share of ATF's budget that is devoted to the enforcement of gun regulations each year, presumably this function would no longer be necessary if guns were no longer subject to misuse.

Finally, law enforcement expenditures throughout the United States would be lower in a number of other ways if gunshot injuries were eliminated. For example, urban police departments may be more likely to assign one rather than two officers per patrol car if the threat of gun violence were eliminated. Police officers might also require less extensive "back up" from other officers in dangerous situations if gunshot injuries were not a concern. And local police departments would probably have to spend less to train, equip, and maintain highly armed tactical units like SWAT teams.

Transportation As anyone who has ever been late for a plane can attest, metal detection and other security precautions impose costs on travelers as well as school children. One study has estimated that the security costs at airports equal around $1.20 per passenger.[13] Assuming that this figure is approximately correct, then the United States spent around $720 million to screen the 598.9 million passengers who were enplaned in 1997.[14] While airports would no doubt continue to screen passengers in some way even if gun violence were no longer a threat, these security expenditures might be lower if gunshot injuries were eliminated, since around one-third of all dangerous articles confiscated by airport security each year are firearms.[15]

Public Housing Public housing agencies across America incur some costs in trying to reduce the prevalence of gun violence and other crimes within the housing complexes that are under their charge. Unfortunately, no systematic data are available on the scope of these expenditures, or on how these costs would be affected by a reduction or elimination of gun violence. Yet there is some indication that these costs may be nontrivial—in the fall of 1999 the U.S. Department of Housing and Urban Development organized a lawsuit against the gun industry on behalf of the nation's 3,200 local public housing authorities, seeking damage claims on the order of $1 billion.[16]

This review suggests that the expenditures of a wide variety of government agencies may be affected by the threat of gun violence in America. Our estimates suggest that government spending on the criminal justice system is around $2 billion higher than it would be in the absence of gun violence. Each year, local police departments spend $100 million on bulletproof vests alone. If the elimination of gun violence enables the government to reduce the Secret Service and ATF budgets by, say, one-quarter, and to reduce the costs of airport screening by one-half, then annual government spending would be reduced by nearly $3 billion. This figure excludes difficult-to-measure savings that would be experienced by schools, public housing agencies, and other government organizations.

Private Prevention Costs

The preventative expenditures made by government agencies are only part of the story, since the behavior of almost every

American is affected in some way by the threat of gun violence. In what follows, we review the different ways in which people incur costs to reduce the risk of gunshot injury. We find that the costs of gun violence from reductions in evening work alone are on the order of $3 to $7 billion each year.

Residential Location

Many of the most striking features of American urban life are so commonplace that they are regularly taken for granted—the exodus of businesses and middle-class residents to the suburbs, increases in traffic congestion and commute times, and deterioration in the economic and social viability of many urban neighborhoods. While these patterns are the result of a complex set of social and political forces, one contributing factor is surely the high rates of gun violence found in our nation's cities.

One of the surprising predictions of urban economics is that gun violence need not lead to suburban flight. The reason is that housing prices in neighborhoods with high rates of gun violence will be depressed by this local disamenity (the heightened threat of being shot). Under certain conditions, the risks of gunshot injury will be capitalized into housing prices to the point where people are indifferent between living in areas with high- versus low-rates of gun violence. In this case, eliminating gun violence may change which people and businesses are located in the city versus the suburbs, but need not affect the population concentration in different parts of the metropolitan area.

In practice, urban housing markets do not appear to work in exactly this way. A study by economists Julie Berry Cullen at the University of Michigan and Steve Levitt at the University of Chicago finds that increases in property and violent crimes on net reduce city populations—suggesting that either the value of local disamenities are not fully capitalized into housing prices, or there are fixed costs of maintaining properties that establish a minimum rent level at which a property can be maintained.[17] Since homicides lead to substantially more suburban flight than other violent crimes, and guns increase the probability that violent crimes result in homicide, the use of guns in crime contributes to suburban flight.

While we cannot readily monetize the costs associated with increased suburban flight, there are reasons to suspect that these costs may be substantial. People's decisions to move to the suburbs may impose a cost on everyone else in the form of increased congestion of local roadways, as well as diminished air quality in the local area. Decisions by firms to relocate to the suburbs may decrease productivity if the clustering together of businesses in the central city increases the productivity of each firm, or reduces the costs of inputs, or both.[18] Suburban flight may also affect the rate of social problems in the central city if middle-class families are more likely than poor families to move in response to increases in gun crime. In his influential 1987 book *The Truly Disadvantaged*, sociologist William Julius Wilson suggested that the flight of middle-class families from urban areas beginning in the 1960s and 1970s in America stripped these neighborhoods of valuable social capital and role models, which in turn increased the likelihood that the low-income families left behind engaged in antisocial behaviors.[19] Some evidence to support Wilson's hypothesis comes from a randomized housing-mobility experiment conducted by the U.S. Department of Housing and Urban Development, which suggests that relocating low-income families from very high- to very low-poverty neighborhoods reduces children's involvement in violent criminal activity by 30 to 50% and adult welfare receipt by around 15%.[20]

Work

The fear of gun violence may also change when and where people are willing to work. Daniel Hamermesh, an economist at the University of Texas at Austin, has demonstrated that each additional homicide in a city prevents between $293,000 and $732,000 worth of night and evening work each year.[21] In contrast, other violent crimes such as robberies and assaults had no effect on off-schedule work. As a result, eliminating gun violence would increase productivity by between $38,000 and

$95,000 per gunshot injury, even if every gun crime were replaced by a nongun crime.[22] These calculations suggest that eliminating all gun assaults in 1997 would increase GNP in the United States by between $3.0 and $7.4 billion just from increases in evening work alone. While it is the share of these additional earnings that are not consumed by workers that is of particular interest to society (Chapter 6), our calculations nevertheless suggest that the effects of gun violence on net production in America could be substantial.

Other Public Activities

Gun violence also imposes costs on society by causing families to stay inside or avoid particular neighborhoods, thereby reducing the overall quality of communal life. Consider, for example, the case of Washington Heights, a neighborhood in New York City where for years people were afraid to venture outside because of the threat of gunfire. One police officer assigned to the area reported that, "We found people who lived across the street from each other for 25 years and had never seen each other." According to one resident, "We were hibernating like bears." Another remarked "I've got to get over my fear. It controls you. It does not allow you to be. It makes you feel like a prisoner when you have not committed a crime."[23] The inability of parents and children to leave their own homes will obviously have substantial negative effects on people's quality of life, even if the dollar value of these costs cannot be readily quantified. In addition to the obvious reductions in recreational and job opportunities that families experience, being homebound may have effects on health outcomes by reducing exercise[24] and trips to the doctor's office, grocery, or drug store.

Even those who live outside of areas with high rates of gun violence may suffer a reduction in their quality of life if the threat of gunshot injury prevents them from taking advantage of the amenities offered by big city life. For example, a friend of ours lives and works in the suburbs of Chicago as an environmental engineer. On several of his business trips to rural areas in Illinois, people have been amazed to learn that he (voluntarily) drives into the city to shop or see White Sox games—"Aren't you afraid of being shot?" is the question he is most frequently asked.[25] The fear of gunshot injury may also increase people's commute times by causing them to take more circuitous routes to work in order to avoid neighborhoods with high rates of gun violence.

Similarly, gun violence may also affect the number of people who visit a metropolitan area as tourists, which also affects economic activity and government revenues. For example, between 1992 and 1993 a total of nine foreign tourists were shot in Miami, Florida, in cases that generated an enormous amount of media attention worldwide. One Miami company reported that the number of Florida tourist packages sold to Europeans in 1993 plummeted by 80% compared with the previous year, and economists estimated that European travel to Florida as a whole during the year would be down by 20%. These reductions may impose real costs on a state whose tourism business generates $30 billion or more each year.[26]

Willingness-to-Pay to Reduce Gun Violence

Our discussion so far points to an apparent paradox. Everyday life in the United States confirms that gun violence is a momentous problem. Yet the dollar figures reported in Chapters 5 and 6 are relatively modest. The answer to this puzzle is that the tangible costs of gun violence, including medical expenditures and lost earnings, are only a small part of the overall problem. The greater part stems from the pain, disability, loss of life, and anguish of friends and family, none of which are reflected in an accounting of tangible losses. Further losses are the result of private and public efforts to prevent or avoid gunshot injuries, as described in Chapter 7. This chapter provides the first attempt to directly measure the comprehensive costs that gun violence imposes on American society using contingent-valuation (cv) survey methods.

Contingent-Valuation

The notion of using contingent-valuation survey methods to estimate what people would pay for small changes in the risk of death or poor health dates back to 1968. Economist Thomas Schelling suggested that in situations where observable market prices are not available for measuring the value of reductions in health risks, "Another way of discovering what the benefits are worth is to ask people."[1] The notion is at odds with the intuition of most economists, who believe that people's actual behavior is a better guide to how they value things than their survey responses to questions about hypothetical behaviors. Nonetheless, Schelling offered a defense for his suggestion:

> It is sometimes argued that asking people is a poor way to find out [about their preferences], because they have no incentive to tell the truth. That is an important point, but hardly decisive. It is also argued, and validly, that people are poor at answering hypothetical questions, especially about important events—that the mood and motive of actual choice are hard to simulate. While this argument casts suspicions on what one finds out by asking questions, it casts suspicion too on those market decisions that involve remote and improbable events. Unexpected death has a hypothetical quality whether it is merely talked about or money is being spent to prevent it.
>
> Asked whether he would buy trip insurance if it were available at the airport (or decline to fly in an aircraft that had a statistically higher accident rate than another if it would save an overnight stop), a man may not give verbally the same answer that his actions in the airport would reveal; he still might not feel that his actual decision was authoritative evidence of his values or that, had mood and circumstance been different—even had the amount of time for consultation and decision been different—his action might have been different too. This problem of coping, as a consumer, with increments in the risk of unexpected death is very much the problem of coping with hypothetical questions, whether in response to survey research or to the man who sells lightning-rod attachments for the TV antenna. If consumers regularly retained professional consultants in coping with such decisions, there might be a good source of information.[2]

Since Schelling's suggestion in 1968, a large literature has developed about how best to implement the cv methodology in practice. This literature has been dominated by environmental economists, who constantly face the problem of determining how the public values changes in a particular public good (environmental quality) that is not traded in the marketplace. For many years, environmental economists toiled away in bliss, using cv methods to estimate the value to society of saving another 50 spotted woodpeckers or cleaning up creeks in North Dakota. And then in March of 1989, the oil tanker *Exxon Valdez* ran aground and spilled 260,000 barrels of oil into Alaska's Prince William Sound.[3]

Public opinion demanded that Exxon be held financially responsible for the damage, but what exactly were the costs of the spill? The financial bill for the oil cleanup would understate the social costs of the accident, since this would ignore the lost recreational opportunities and damage to the local ecosystem, including the death of between 260,000 and 580,000 birds.[4] In an attempt to estimate the value to society of a clean Prince William's Sound, state and federal governments reportedly spent almost $7 million (in 1998 dollars) for contingent-valuation studies.[5] Yet the government money spent on CV research was the least of it. The enormous financial damages that were at stake, together with most people's natural suspicion of responses to surveys, motivated Exxon to fund a number of prominent economists to reexamine the reliability of CV methods. The result has been an ongoing debate about the value of contingent valuation, which in turn has produced much useful information about the method.

In an attempt to synthesize what had been learned and to determine whether CV studies had any merit at all for public policy, the National Oceanic and Atmospheric Administration (NOAA) convened a blue-ribbon panel in 1992 chaired by Nobel laureate Kenneth Arrow of Stanford University. The NOAA panel outlined the key components of a CV study that would maximize the likelihood of producing reliable results,[6] which include the use of a referendum format that asks respondents to vote on a hypothetical government program. The referendum format is deemed preferable to open-ended questions because citizens have experience in casting such votes and because the referendum format minimizes incentives to "free ride"—that is, report low values because the respondent knows that other citizens will be willing to bear the financial burden of providing the good.[7] Other desirable attributes for CV studies include the use of random probability samples (rather than samples of convenience), scenarios that are realistic and comprehensible, reminders that funds devoted to the hypothetical good in question could not be devoted to other uses, follow-up questions to ensure that the respondents understood the cv questions, and, where possible, in-person rather than telephone surveys, and telephone surveys rather than self-administered mail surveys.[8]

Even if these ideal conditions can be met, the reliability of cv estimates rests on a number of assumptions. As with studies of wage-risk tradeoffs, cv estimates will only be reliable if respondents understand the baseline risks and how they are changed by the particular intervention that is being asked about. In studies of wage-risk tradeoffs, economists typically assume that people will seek out information about health risks on their own, since they have strong incentives to do so. With cv studies that examine unusual health risks to which most people are typically not exposed, the only information that respondents may have about the nature of the risk is what is provided to them as part of the survey. This concern should be less of an issue with our study of gun violence, since the threat of gunshot injury affects people's everyday behaviors—for example, decisions about where to live and when and where to work.[9] Because people have incentives to acquire information about the risks of gun violence on their own, respondents should be less dependent on the survey interviewer for information about the baseline risks of gunshot injury.

Contingent-valuation researchers must also hope that respondents provide thoughtful answers to survey questions about the public good in question, that are guided by the respondent's preferences for the particular good that will be provided. Economists are typically less concerned with what motivates actual consumer decisions in the marketplace, since people have incentives to devote at least some reflection to their decisions (since their money and, in some cases, health are at stake). To maximize the chance that respondents take the contingent-valuation questions seriously, high-quality studies make the hypothetical market scenario as realistic as possible and precede the cv segment with a sequence of questions that get the respondent thinking about the public good of interest. There is, of course, no guarantee that these efforts will be successful.

Another potential problem arises from the well-known tendency of survey respondents to try to present themselves favorably to interviewers, which produces what is known as "social desirability bias" or "yea-saying."[10] Since most contingent-valuation surveys ask about public goods that most people would deem to be socially desirable—whales, open meadows, better health for the community's children—respondents may report to the interviewer that they will pay to support these good causes, even if they would refuse to pay in a real-life situation. A similar problem comes from the potential desire of some respondents to answer in ways that they themselves think are socially desirable, so that the respondent's answers are motivated more by a desire to purchase "moral satisfaction" rather than a defined quantity of the specific public good in question.[11] These alternative motivations may manifest themselves in what is known as the "embedding effect," where the amount that the respondent is willing to pay is independent of the quantity of the public good that is being provided. (An example of the embedding effect is when people will pay the same amount to save 5,000 seals as 5,000,000 seals.)

What is the evidence for the embedding effect in practice? Most studies find some relationship between the quantity or scope of the public good being asked about and the amount that respondents will pay.[12] Two noteworthy exceptions[13] understandably make skeptics nervous about the cv method, though cv proponents argue that these studies use unreliable survey methods and thus do not provide a fair test of the embedding phenomenon.[14] Whether people's wtp responses change *enough* in response to changes in the quantity of the public good being offered remains the subject of a highly technical debate.[15]

More general tests of the reliability of the contingent-valuation method come from comparing the results of cv surveys with people's actual behavior. Most studies that compare what people report they will pay to support environmental goods (like public parks) with their actual behavior apparently find quite close agreement.[16] On the other hand, mixed results are obtained by controlled randomized experiments, which show agreement between cv reports and actual behavior in about half of all studies,[17] though proponents of cv argue that the studies showing disagreement between reported and actual behavior use low-quality surveying methods and poorly designed questions.[18]

In sum, most economists agree that willingness-to-pay is the conceptually appropriate way to define the value of some public good (such as a reduction in gun violence), though there remains some disagreement about whether contingent-valuation surveys can reliably measure these values. Our own view is that contingent valuation is, for all its problems, at least as useful as extrapolating from studies of marketplace behavior and jury awards, as is commonly done within health economics.[19] The two approaches share many similar assumptions about the preferences, information, and rationality of consumers; while studies of workplace behavior have the advantage of relying on actual rather than hypothetical behaviors, contingent-valuation methods will in principle be more complete. The next section describes our attempt to estimate the costs of gun violence using this contingent-valuation approach.

Willingness-To-Pay Estimates

In 1998, the Joyce Foundation and the Johns Hopkins Center for Gun Policy and Research sponsored a national telephone survey that included a sequence of questions that asked respondents what they would pay to reduce the volume of gunshot injuries from assault. These survey data meet many, but not all, of the ideal conditions for contingent-valuation estimation outlined by the NOAA blue-ribbon panel. The results suggest that the American public is willing to pay on the order of $24 billion to reduce gun assaults by 30%. If reductions in preventative expenditures are proportional to reductions in gunshot injuries, our figures suggest that eliminating the use of guns in assault would produce benefits of perhaps $80 billion or more to the American public, or roughly $1 million per gunshot injury. While the CV data used in these analyses have some limitations, the resultant estimates are generally consistent with a number of reasonable benchmarks.

Data

Our data come from a nationally representative telephone survey of 1,204 American adults in fall 1998 called the National Gun Policy Survey (NGPS). The NGPS was conducted by the National Opinion Research Center (NORC) at the University of Chicago, one of the country's leading survey organizations. Within each sampled household, one adult was chosen at random to be interviewed. The response rate for the NGPS was 61%.[20]

After a series of questions asking about their attitudes toward government and various current or proposed gun regulations, respondents are asked: "Suppose that you were asked to vote for or against a new program in your state to reduce gun thefts and illegal gun dealers. This program would make it more difficult for criminals and delinquents to obtain guns. It would reduce gun injuries by about 30% but taxes would have to be increased to pay for it. If it would cost you an extra [$50 / $100 / $200] in annual taxes would you vote for or against this new program?" The amount of the tax increase that the respondent is asked about, either $50, $100 or $200, is randomly determined by the survey software, so that answers for each of the three dollar amounts are available from around one-third of the sample. Respondents are then asked a follow-up where the dollar amount asked about in the initial referendum question is either doubled or halved, depending on whether the respondent's initial answer was positive or negative, respectively.

Thus, respondents are being asked to report on WTP to fund a program that decreases gun availability to proscribed groups at high risk of misusing firearms (teens and convicted felons) while having little effect on access to guns by ordinary citizens. Previous research suggests that gun availability within an area increases the lethality but not the volume of violent crime (Chapter 3). As a result, the implicit counterfactual that we have in mind is a reduction in assault-related gunshot injuries by 30%, an equivalent increase in nongun crimes, and no change in the number of defensive gun uses by law-abiding citizens. It is possible that respondents ignore the possibility of a countervailing increase in nongun crimes when formulating their WTP responses, which will lead them to overstate the value of moving from the *status quo* to the counterfactual that we have in mind. Yet the degree of bias is likely to be modest, given that Americans appear to be far more worried about serious injuries than about other criminal victimizations. For example, as noted in Chapter 7, Daniel Hamermesh finds that the amount of evening work in a metropolitan area is affected by the rate of homicides (the majority of which involve firearms), but not by the rates of violent crimes that do not result in the victim's death.[21] Similarly, Julie Cullen and Steve Levitt find that each additional homicide causes a city's population to decrease by 70 people from suburban flight, while each nonfatal violent crime causes only a one-person reduction in city population.[22]

We also assume that respondents are reporting on the total dollar value that their *household* would be willing to pay to fund this program, rather than reporting strictly on the value that they themselves would pay.[23] Our assumption is conservative in that if respondents are in fact reporting on personal rather than household WTP, our estimates will understate total societal WTP to fund the hypothetical reduction in gun crime.[24]

Nonparametric Estimates

Table 8.1 presents the descriptive statistics from the NGPS data. The proportion of respondents who vote to support the violence-reduction program decreases as the amount required to fund the program increases, ranging from 76% at a cost of $50 more in annual taxes to 38% at a cost of $400.

Figure 8.1 provides a graphical representation of the proportion of people who are willing to support the program at different prices implied by these descriptive statistics. This fig-

Table 8.1
Descriptive Statistics from the 1998 National Gun Policy Survey

	How would you vote on a program to reduce gunshot injuries by 30% that cost $50 more per year in income taxes?	How would you vote on a program to reduce gunshot injuries by 30% that cost $100 more per year in income taxes?	How would you vote on a program to reduce gunshot injuries by 30% that cost $200 more per year in income taxes?
Percentage voting in favor of program (N)	75.8 (400)	68.5 (400)	63.6 (404)
Amount asked about on follow-up question			
$25	23.3 (95)		
$50		24.2 (112)	
$100	67.2 (290)		27.9 (133)
$200		59.4 (268)	
$400			59.4 (253)

Source: Authors' calculations from 1998 NGPS; descriptive statistics are calculated using the 1998 NGPS sampling weights. Figures are in 1998 dollars.

ure (known as a cumulative distribution function in statistics) is not unlike a demand curve, in the sense that the graph shows the proportion of households that are willing to "purchase" (vote for) a 30% reduction in gun assaults at each possible "price" (tax increase).

The cumulative distribution function presented in Figure 8.1 can be used to calculate what the American public would pay to reduce gun assaults by 30%. If we integrate under the area shown in Figure 8.1 (that is, sum up the area under the curve) and multiply by the total number of households in the United States—equal to 99.6 million in 1996[25]—we obtain an estimated total WTP of $21.2 billion to reduce assault-related gunshot injuries by 30% (Table 8.2.) In these calculations, we assign a WTP

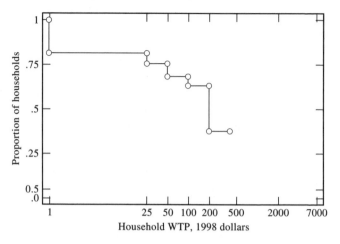

Figure 8.1 Cumulative Distribution: Willingness to Pay to Reduce Gun Violence 30%. 1998 National Gun Policy Survey, National Opinion Research Center, University of Chicago.

of $0 to those respondents who answer no to both the first and follow-up cv questions, under the assumption that each individual's wtp to reduce gunshot injuries must be nonnegative. While some people may object to the specific *mechanism* used to reduce gun injuries, presumably few people would be willing to pay to see more Americans shot, and in any case it is not clear that such preferences should be given standing in benefit-cost analyses. These estimates are what economists call "nonparametric" in the sense that they impose almost no assumptions on how wtp is distributed across households and are entirely data-driven.

In addition to an estimate for the total value of reducing gun assaults by 30%, we are interested in obtaining a nonparametric estimate for wtp per gunshot injury avoided. We divide the total wtp by the estimated annual incidence of assault-related gunshot woundings (77,923 in 1997, as shown in Table 2.1) multiplied by 30%. This suggests wtp per injury equal to around $900,000.

Table 8.2
Nonparametric Estimates for Mean WTP from NGPS

Frequency distribution of maxiumum WTP to reduce gun assaults by 30% implied by descriptive statistics in Table 1	(% households)
$ 0	18.6
25	5.6
50	7.3
100	4.9
200	25.8
400	37.8
Mean WTP per household to reduce assault-related gun violence by 30%	$212.7
Total societal WTP to reduce assault-related gun violence by 30%[a]	$21.2 billion
Implied WTP per assault-related gunshot injury[b]	$906,874

Notes: Estimates calculated from (weighted) descriptive statistics for NGPS shown in Table 1. Results reported in 1998 dollars.

[a] Obtained by multiplying mean WTP per household by number of households in United States in 1996, which is equal to 99.6 million (U.S. Bureau of the Census, 1997).

[b] Calculated by dividing total societal WTP by the 0.3 times the number of assault-related gunshot injuries in the United States in 1997 (equal to 77,923, as shown in Table 2.1).

Parametric Estimates

The nonparametric estimate may understate societal WTP because it does not interpolate the underlying distribution ("demand curve") between the CV bid values, or extrapolate beyond the highest value used in the survey. The nonparametric approach is also limited in that it only uses a fraction of the information available with the CV data. In this section, we present refined estimates that use maximum-likelihood methods to estimate societal WTP under a number of different assumptions. These estimates are "parametric" in that these assumptions impose some structure on the shape of the distribution of WTP.

While the technical details of our approach are relegated to Appendix D, the general intuition is relatively straightforward: by making some assumptions about the shape of the distribution of WTP across households, we can smooth the curve between the survey's bid values and extrapolate beyond the highest bid value that is asked about in the survey. Our starting assumption is that the natural logarithm of each household's willingness-to-pay has a normal ("bell-shaped") distribution. This assumption yields estimates that imply a new demand curve as shown in Figure 8.2, which is overlaid against the nonparametric curve for comparison. This new demand curve implies that the average household in America will pay around $200 to reduce gun assaults by 30%, which implies a total societal WTP equal to around $20 billion, or around $860,000 per gunshot injury (Table 8.3.) The parametric estimate does not exceed the nonparametric figure as might be expected because the former uses data from both the first and second CV questions, while the latter is based largely on responses to the first CV question.

We can further refine these parametric estimates by calculating mean household WTP controlling for a set of household characteristics that may affect the risk of gunshot injury, atti-

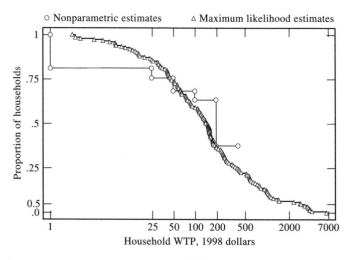

Figure 8.2. Cumulative Distribution: Willingness to Pay to Reduce Gun Violence 30%, Nonparametric and Maximum Likelihood Estimates. 1992 National Gun Policy Survey, National Opinion Research Center, University of Chicago.

Table 8.3

Parametric Maximum Likelihood Estimates for WTP to Reduce Gun Assaults by 30%, from NGPS Data

	Without covariates	With covariates[c]
Estimated willingness-to-pay per household to reduce GSW by 30%		
Mean	$203	$239
(95% confidence interval)	(185–220)	(103–375)
Median	$203	$204
(95% confidence interval)	(185–220)	(68–340)
Total societal WTP to reduce assault-related gun violence by 30%[a]	$20.2 billion	$23.8 billion
Implied WTP per assault-related gunshot injury[b]	$864,097	$1,018,095

Notes: Figures are in 1998 dollars.

[a] Obtained by multiplying mean WTP per household by number of households in United States in 1996, which is equal to 99.6 million (U.S. Bureau of the Census, 1997).

[b] Calculated by dividing total societal WTP by the 0.3 times the number of assault-related gunshot injuries in the United States in 1997 (equal to 77,923, as shown in Table 2.1).

[c] Covariates included in model are household income, household composition (the number of children under 6 or 6 to 17, and the number of adults), household gun ownership status, and race.

tudes toward risk, or ability to pay. The household characteristics that we control for include income, household composition (the number of children under 6 or 6 to 17, and the number of adults), household gun ownership, and race.[26] As shown in Appendix D, the correlations between these household characteristics and the probability of supporting the program are of the expected signs, thus providing some support for the credibility of the underlying survey responses. For example, household income has a strong positive effect on support for the violence program, and households with guns are less likely to support the program. We also find that what respondents will pay to reduce gun violence increases with the number of children in the home, providing some support for the idea that respondents are reporting household (rather than individual) willingness-to-pay.

Including the household covariates serves to increase our estimated mean WTP per household from $203 to $239 (Table 8.3.) Total WTP to reduce gun violence by 30% equals $23.8 billion, or around $1 million per injury.

If a 30% reduction in gun assaults leads to a 30% reduction in preventative expenditures, then our estimates imply that eliminating gun use in assault would be worth nearly $80 billion. Since averting behavior may not be proportional to the volume of gun violence, and in fact many preventive activities may only be avoided with a complete elimination of gunshot injuries, our calculations for the value of eliminating all gunshot injuries are only a rough lower bound for the true figure. As discussed in Appendix D, our estimates are generally robust to our decisions about how to estimate the model.

What Do These Estimates Mean?

The most fundamental issue is whether these survey responses reflect respondents' preferences about a given quantity of violence reduction rather than social desirability bias, moral satisfaction, or some other motivation. CV responses that are motivated by something other than the public's demand for a public good may be insensitive to the quantity of the public good that is offered (the embedding effect) and thus will not be useful for benefit-cost analysis.

One crude test for an embedding effect with these data suggests that WTP is in fact sensitive to the amount of risk reduction provided. We show in Appendix D that WTP increases with the number of children in the home, which in turn is related to the total amount of risk reduction that the household gains from a violence-reduction program. Since these findings could be explained by taste or other differences between households with and without children, we reestimated our models using only those households with children. We find that each additional child in the home under the age of six increases the respondent's WTP by 50%, and each additional child between 6 and 17 increases WTP by 25%. While these findings provide some evidence against an embedding effect, for some reason household WTP does not appear to increase with the number of adults within the home.

Another potential concern with these estimates arises if the risks of gun violence are at least partially capitalized into local housing prices. In this case, landlords may bear part of the victimization costs of renters in the form of decreases in producer surplus, and what renters will pay to reduce their risks of injury may be reduced by this amount.[27] One implication is that if CV surveys fail to capture what landlords will pay to reduce gun violence in the areas around their rental properties, the result will be an underestimate of what society would pay to reduce or eliminate gunshot injuries (as might occur if, for example, a CV question asks respondents what they would pay for reductions in risk only in their local community). This measurement problem is mitigated to some extent with the NGPS, since respondents are asked about the value of programs that have state-level impacts. Yet the capitalization of the risks of gun violence in housing rents has distributional implications as well—the possibility that landlords bear part of the victimization costs of renters provides another reason why the costs of gun violence are distributed more evenly across society than victimization statistics would suggest.

A larger concern is that these CV data are limited in a number of ways by the constraints of telephone survey methods—respondents are only willing to stay on the telephone for so long, and questions must be simple enough so that they can be easily followed over the phone. The CV questions included in the NGPS can be criticized for excluding important information about the hypothetical interventions that respondents are asked to support, a problem that plagues all CV studies to some degree. The NGPS questions also do not specify the baseline risk of injury to respondents, or the actual change in risk that the respondent experiences, even though the heterogeneity in the risk of gunshot injury within the population implies that a 30% reduction in risk will mean different things for different respondents. A related concern is that the questions do not specify where the interventions will be targeted, and thus who will benefit from the program. For example, what society will pay to reduce gun injuries to elementary-school children may be different from what society will pay to reduce the number of gang shootings.

Despite these limitations, our estimates imply a value per statistical life that is remarkably consistent with what is found from previous studies of wage-risk tradeoffs in the labor market. Deriving the value per statistical life that is implied by our CV results is complicated by the fact that these CV responses reflect willingness-to-pay for both fatal and nonfatal gunshot injuries. If we start with the extreme assumption that WTP is driven entirely by concern about fatal gunshot injuries, then since around one-fifth of gunshot injuries are fatal, our preferred estimate of around $1 million per gunshot injury implies a value per statistical life of $5 million. This estimate fits comfortably within the range of values for a statistical life that have been estimated from marketplace behavior, equal to between $3.7 and $8.6 million.[28]

Since presumably part of what people will pay to reduce gun violence is motivated by concern about nonfatal injuries, our CV data will imply a value per statistical life that is somewhat less than $5 million. If we (arbitrarily) assume that nonfatal gunshot injuries are twice as undesirable as the average workplace injury, our CV estimates imply a value per statistical life of around $3.8 million.[29]

Another useful check is to compare what the average household will pay to reduce gun violence by 30% (which we have estimated to be between $200 and $240 per year) with what the average household currently pays to avoid criminal victimization. National estimates calculated by economist David Anderson[30] suggest that each year the American public devotes $174.6 billion to reduce the risk of criminal victimization through spending on the criminal justice system and private protective measures such as home security systems or protective fences, equal to nearly $1,800 per year per household. Thus, it does not seem implausible that the average household will spend around $200 more per year to reduce the risk of gun violence by 30%. This is particularly true in light of the arguments made by criminologists Franklin Zimring and Gordon Hawkins that the fear of crime in America is driven largely by the fear of *violent* crime,[31] a hypothesis that receives some support from the Hamermesh and Cullen/Levitt studies mentioned earlier.[32]

Finally, we can compare our contingent-valuation estimates with the results obtained from extrapolating from studies of marketplace behavior and jury awards (discussed in detail in Appendix D). As we have argued above, such extrapolations have the disadvantage of excluding the value of what people will pay for reductions in risk to those they care about, as well as for reductions in preventative expenditures. These alternative estimates suggest a WTP to eliminate gun assaults in 1997 of between $6 and $60 billion.[33]

Distribution of Costs

In Chapters 5 and 6, we demonstrated that the direct costs of gun violence in America from increased medical expenditures and lost productivity is less than $1 billion per year. The real costs of gun violence, we have argued, come from the devastating emotional costs experienced by relatives and friends of gunshot victims, and the fear and general reduction in quality of life that the threat of gun violence imposes on everyone in America, including people who are not victimized.

The contingent-valuation estimates that we present here suggest that the American public would pay on the order of $80 billion per year to eliminate the use of guns in violent crimes, given the volume of gun violence observed in 1997. While our estimates may be subject to some error for a number of reasons, these calculations clearly demonstrate that the costs of gun violence to society are orders of magnitude larger than the tangible costs from medical spending and productivity losses.

Another striking finding is that the costs of gun violence are distributed far more evenly than what is suggested by statistics on who gets shot. Chapter 2 demonstrated that while everyone in the United States is at some risk for gunshot injury, these risks are concentrated among the poor. Gun assaults in particular are strongly concentrated among low-income young men. Yet our contingent-valuation survey suggests that what households will pay to reduce the volume of gun assaults in America *increases* with family income, even though higher-income families are at lower risk of injury.

If people's support for efforts to reduce gun violence were motivated purely by concern about their own personal safety, we would have expected the public's willingness-to-pay to be far less than $1 million per gunshot assault. The reason is that the people who are at relatively high risk of being injured apparently do not put a high value on reductions in these risks. For example, economist Steve Levitt and sociologist Sudhir Venkatesh studied the records documenting the opportunities and violence-victimization risks for members of a crack-dealing street gang: comparing the risk to the reward suggests that they placed a value on a statistical life of just $55,000 on average.[34] However, the people who place a relatively high value on improvements in their own personal safety are at relatively low risk. The implication is that a large share of the costs of gun violence to America each year stem from interdependencies among people—most people are risk averse and at low risk of gunshot injury themselves, but suffer real costs when people within their social network or their community more generally are shot. In principle, these contingent-valuation estimates may also capture the value that people place on reductions in preventative behaviors within the community, although in practice a 30% reduction in gun assaults may have more modest proportional effects on avoidance costs. Thus, our cv estimates suggesting that the public would pay $80 billion to eliminate gun assaults is probably a lower-bound for the true value.

Because the contingent-valuation survey data used in this chapter only ask respondents about their willingness to pay to reduce gun use in crime, we cannot develop cv estimates for the value of reductions in unintentional shootings or suicides. More generally, thinking about what people would pay to reduce their risks of self-inflicted gun injuries, as with suicide, raises difficult questions about the conditions under which public policies should be responsive to people's preferences and how to identify someone's "true" preferences. Since many of those who survive a suicide attempt do not attempt to injure themselves again,[35] there appears to be some element of impulsiveness or regret associated with at least some self-inflicted injuries. We think about people's willingness to pay in this case as the value of some intervention that reduces the risk that someone will injure themselves in the future in response to such an impulse.[36] Using data from workplace studies and jury awards for the value per statistical life and nonfatal injury, we estimate that the elimination of unintentional shootings and gun suicides in 1997 would be worth as much as $20 billion (Appendix D). Taken together, the best available evidence suggests that the costs of gun violence in America are on the order of $100 billion per year, plus the value of the avoidance and prevention behaviors discussed in Chapter 7.

9

Remedies

We have demonstrated that the costs of gun violence in the United States are enormous, on the order of $100 billion per year, and affect all of our lives in countless ways. Gun violence devastates families and draws tax revenues away from other pressing social problems. The threat of gunshot injury causes people to be fearful for their own safety as well as for their loved ones, which in turn distorts our decisions about where we work, live, shop, and go to school, and changes our behavior in other ways that reduce our quality of life.

What, then, should be done? Perhaps the least controversial approach has been to deter gun use in crime through the threat of harsher penalties. In most states, a robber who uses a gun is subject to an "enhancement" in the prison sentence, and in some jurisdictions criminals arrested with a gun in their possession may be prosecuted in federal court where the prison sentences tend to be longer than in state courts. More controversial by far have been policies that are traditionally included under the "gun control" rubric, policies that limit who may acquire a gun in the first place and what kinds of guns and ammunition are permitted in commerce. A third approach is to limit the more dangerous uses of guns, and particularly the practice of carrying a gun in public; in recent years a number of city police departments have begun patrolling against illicit carrying, while a majority of states have actually loosened the laws restricting who has a right to carry a concealed gun.

It is plausible that all of these approaches have the potential of reducing gun violence and hence the homicide rate. The empirical evidence on the effectiveness of such policies is not as strong as we might like, but dispassionate observers will learn something from a close look at the evidence on what "works" in reducing gun use in violence.

Interventions

Our topic is those strategies for reducing gun use in crime that are intended to work *not* by reducing crime, but by reducing gun use in crime. We have demonstrated in earlier chapters that guns are more lethal than other weapons typically used to commit crimes, and as a result, a decrease in the share of crimes committed with guns will save lives. So will measures that are effective in reducing unintentional discharges, or, possibly, in keeping guns away from despondent youths or others at high risk of an impulsive suicide attempt.

The heart of the policy response to gun violence focuses on efforts to reduce gun use in crime by restricting supply and thus making it more difficult, time consuming, or costly for a violent individual to obtain a gun. We begin our discussion with this approach, and then go on to discuss other efforts to reduce gun misuse.

Acquisition

Whether violent people can be disarmed through restricting the supply of guns remains a topic of debate. The backbone of current efforts to regulate gun acquisitions are prohibitions against the sale of guns by federally licensed firearm dealers (FFLS) to people prohibited from owning a gun, including teenagers, convicted felons, fugitives from justice, and those with serious mental illnesses. FFLS are also required to conduct background checks on prospective buyers to enforce these restrictions.

In reality, there are ways around these various prohibitions and restrictions, and as a result the change in the effective price of guns to teens and criminals are likely to be modest. One concern about supply-side strategies is that they only apply to sales that involve FFLS, which constitute the "primary market." Left largely unregulated are the 30 to 40% of all gun sales that do not involve an FFL, so-called "secondary market" sales.[1] The seller in these cases may be an uncle or next-door neighbor, but may also be someone in the business of trafficking guns illegally or an acquaintance who makes a straw purchase from an FFL for someone who can't pass the background check. While many secondary-market transactions are innocent and legal, most of the transactions that supply guns for teens and convicted felons are in this market.[2]

Despite the presence of an active secondary market in guns, regulations of primary-market sales have the potential to affect proscribed individuals in several ways. First, in the absence of primary-market regulations that ban the sale of guns to high-risk individuals and require background checks to enforce this ban, some teenagers and criminals would acquire guns directly from gun dealers in the primary market. Because of primary-market regulations, many of these buyers are forced into the secondary market, where the dollar price of guns is in some areas higher than the price of a similar gun in the primary market.[3] The secondary market is also less convenient and entails greater risks—a gun purchased from a stranger may be damaged or "have a body on it" (that is, the gun may have been used by a previous owner to commit a homicide).

Second, the influx of additional buyers into the secondary market caused by primary-market regulations will, under standard supply-demand analysis, further increase the price of guns in the secondary market. This additional increase in the price of guns will cause further reductions in gun ownership by high-risk groups on the margin.

Third, other regulations may increase the price of guns in the secondary market by reducing the flow of guns from the primary to the secondary market. For example, three states now restrict handgun sales to no more than one per customer per month, thus making life more difficult for illicit gun traffickers. Evidence that such restrictions reduce gun trafficking comes from a study by Doug Weil and Rebecca Knox, who find that the proportion of crime guns in the Northeast that are traced to dealers in Virginia (a state with relatively lax gun laws) decreased by 30% after implementation of that state's one-gun-a-month law.[4]

Any change in the effective price of guns to high-risk people will reduce gun ownership among such groups so long as at least some members are sensitive to the cost of acquiring and keeping firearms. Available evidence supports the notion that the demand for guns by high-risk groups is not entirely inelastic. In a survey of incarcerated juveniles in North Carolina, one teen reported that "When [people] are short on money, they have no choice but to sell [their guns]," while another remarked that he had "traded a .22 for a Super Nintendo and some other guns for a VCR and for my waterbed. I got other stuff for my room, like a phone with lights and a copy [fax] machine for a twenty-gauge."[5] Similarly, in a survey of incarcerated felons who committed their crimes without guns, 21% reported that the trouble of acquiring a gun was somewhat or very important in their decision not to use a gun, while 17% reported "cost" as a somewhat or very important consideration.[6] The implication is that while highly motivated teens and criminals may not be deterred from acquiring guns, increases in the price of guns to proscribed groups should reduce gun ownership at the margin.

A final group of high-risk individuals who may be deterred by primary-market regulations are those who have some passing impulse to acquire and misuse a gun. For example, the 1994 Brady Act required a five-day waiting period for all handgun sales in order to provide a "cooling off" period for crimes of passion or temporary rage, and to deter temporarily distraught individuals from shooting themselves. That provision was sunsetted in 1998, but waiting periods remain in place in many states.

None of the policies mentioned here are likely to have any substantial effect on the ability of law-abiding citizens to acquire guns for the purposes of recreation or protection. Some people who urgently need a gun for protection may be affected by waiting periods, but that is a minor exception to the rule. So even if primary-market regulations achieve only modest reductions in the homicide or suicide rate, that may be sufficient to compensate for the modest burden imposed on law-abiding adults.

Here we consider three approaches that have been subjected to evaluation: background checks, handgun bans, and gun buy-back programs.

Background Checks Do background checks on would-be handgun buyers have any effect? A study of individual California gun buyers by Mona Wright, Garen Wintemute, and Frederick Rivara suggest that they do, although it is modest.[7] Wright and colleagues compared Californians who tried to purchase a handgun but were denied because of a prior felony conviction in 1977 with those who had a prior felony arrest but were allowed to purchase because they had not been convicted. The "denied" group had more serious criminal records on the average and hence would be expected to be a greater continuing threat to the community. But Wright found that during the first three years after the purchase attempts the "arrest only" group had 21% more gun arrests and 24% more violent-crime arrests than those denied purchase. It thus appears that the denial had some effect on the likelihood that the felons acquired a gun. Still, the effect of these denials on gun injuries appears to be relatively small, since the convicted felons who try to obtain guns from licensed dealers have relatively low rates of criminal involvement.[8]

The evidence presented by Wright provides no indication of how the background-screening requirement affects felons and other proscribed groups who do not attempt to purchase a gun from a dealer. If some are discouraged from acquiring a gun, then the logical result could be to render them less of a threat to the community, but also more vulnerable to attack by their enemies.

Some evidence on the overall effects of such policies comes from an evaluation of the 1994 Brady Law, which required background checks and a five-day waiting period for all handgun sales by licensed gun dealers in the 32 states that did not have such provisions already in place. A comparison of homicide trends in the "Brady" and "Brady exempt" states found little or no difference.[9] This finding does not mean that screening primary-market sales is of no consequence for gun violence. Brady may have had some indirect effect on gun violence in the "Brady-exempt" states by reducing gun-running across state lines.[10] And even before Brady went into effect, federal law required FFLS to check identification and keep a record on each sale, which as we have seen is sufficient to divert most felons and teenagers from the primary market.

The effects of primary-market gun regulations surely depend on the extent to which the secondary market in guns is regulated. The current system leaves secondary market sales largely unregulated, thereby providing an enormous loophole that works to limit the effectiveness of primary-market regulations.

Handgun Ban A more extreme example of primary-market regulation is the 1976 ban on the purchase, sale, transfer, and possession of handguns in Washington, D.C. While a national ban on handguns is unlikely in the foreseeable future, examining Washington's ban provides useful information about the effects of primary-market regulations, since the ban increases the price of guns to teens and convicted criminals by forcing them to either use the secondary market or drive to Virginia or Maryland to attempt to buy guns (illegally) from licensed dealers. In principle, the effects of this law on gun violence are ambiguous, since the ban also raises the price of guns to law-abiding citizens who seek guns for self-protection. And some have argued that handgun restrictions may lead criminals to substitute long guns, which are more lethal than handguns, rather than knives, fists, or baseball bats, which are less lethal.[11] Yet an evaluation of the law by criminologist Colin Loftin and his colleagues provides some evidence that the net effect of the handgun ban was to reduce gun violence.[12]

Everyone agrees that gun homicides and suicides decreased by around 25% in the years following Washington's handgun ban. What remains controversial is how much of this reduction to attribute to the handgun ban rather than other causes. Loftin found that gun violence in Washington fell in comparison with gun violence in its suburbs. While Loftin's choice of a "control group" has been criticized, given the obvious socioeconomic differences between the city and the suburbs, comparisons with other jurisdictions tend to reinforce the original findings.[13,14] Taken together, these findings provide some additional support for our view that supply-side strategies can reduce gun violence.

Gun Buybacks In 1999, President Clinton earmarked $15 million dollars for gun buy-back programs. This federal program is based on a number of local initiatives that attempt to reduce the supply of guns in an area by purchasing guns from private citizens on a "no questions asked" basis. Proponents of these measures are persuaded by case-control findings that gun ownership is a risk factor for suicide or unintentional fatal injuries, and thus hope that gun buyback programs can save lives by reducing the proportion of households that keep guns. While that may be true, the results are likely to be trivial in a context where 40 million households own guns and 4 million new guns are added to this private inventory each year.

Gun buyback programs may also have unintended consequences. In order for such programs to attract guns from people who were not planning to dispose of them already, the buy-back price must be high enough to lure guns away from the prospective owners and potential secondary-market buyers. For example, the city of Washington paid $100 per gun as part of its 1999 buy-back program, yet many of the guns that were turned in were estimated to have resale values of no more than $30.[15] The difference enabled at least some owners to upgrade to newer and more lethal firearms, as suggested by the posting of one program participant to an MSNBC electronic bulletin board: "[The D.C. gun buy-back program] gave me an idea, being a gun owner and all, so guess what I did a little while ago?—Yep, I turned in a whole passel of hardware to our dear ole'[government]. I spent the previous two years collecting all the junk, nonfiring, worthless examples of the modern firearm and turned them all in. (Really—none were repairable!) I made nearly six grand on the deal. With the proceeds, I turned around and bought (yes, bought!) some really serious hardware that actually will fire if it becomes necessary to test out some ammunition now and then. . . . The city of D.C. paid for a bunch of new guns, and I didn't pay anything but a few dollars here and there for junk."[16]

Gun Use

Government efforts to reduce gun misuse include the regulation of activities that are relevant to the risk of injury, including gun carrying and storage, as well as sentencing enhancements to discourage the use of guns in crime. The available empirical evidence on these policies is more reliable than what is available for regulations of gun acquisitions, which enables us to take the next step and begin to consider relative benefits and costs.

Carrying Even if the regulatory apparatus fails and dangerous people succeed in acquiring guns, it may still be possible to discourage them from carrying those guns into public places. Some evidence for the effectiveness of police patrols to combat illegal gun carrying comes from the Kansas City Gun Experiment, in which the police department stepped up patrols to target gun carrying in one high-crime area of the city but not in another area that had a similar number of drive-by shootings at baseline.[17] While the treatment area experienced a 49% reduction in gun crimes during the study period, gun crimes increased by 4% in the comparison area during this period and decreased by only 2% in Kansas City as a whole. Since there is no guarantee that the trends in crime in the two areas would have been identical in the absence of the intervention, particularly because there are some differences in crime trends during the preintervention period between the two neighborhoods, it is difficult to determine how much of the reduction in gun crimes in the treatment area can be attributed to the program. Evidence that there was a substantial difference in the numbers of guns seized by police in the treatment versus control area suggests that at least part of the difference may have been due to the gun patrols.[18]

The costs of the Kansas City intervention in the form of the additional police time required to implement the program was around $180,000.[19] Other costs are also relevant, such as the costs to the innocent citizens who are stopped as part of these patrols, though the dollar value of these cannot be readily quantified. On the other side, the benefits from the Kansas City gun experiment may be enormous. If we assume that the entire difference in gun crimes between the treatment and control areas was due to the intervention, then the benefits of the program are on the order of $22 to $100 million.

Safe Storage Keeping guns stored safely locked and unloaded is encouraged by most gun groups to prevent unintentional injury to children. Yet many gun owners apparently believe that keeping a gun stored safely impedes the value of the gun in defense against a criminal attack, as evidenced by the fact that 57% of all handguns are usually kept unlocked, 55% are kept loaded, and 34% are kept both unlocked and loaded.[20]

In order to provide owners with additional incentives to keep guns stored safely, between 1989 and 1993 a total of 12 states enacted laws that make it a criminal offense to store guns in a manner that makes them accessible to children. Peter Cummings and his colleagues at the University of Washington evaluated the effects of these laws on unintentional shootings to children under 15 over the period 1979 through 1994, controlling for state population characteristics (age, sex, and race), national trends, and unobserved fixed differences across states in the rate of unintentional shootings.[21] The authors find that in the three states that allowed for a felony prosecution of parents who store their guns unsafely (California, Connecticut, and Florida), the number of unintentional shootings decreased by 41%. However, in the remaining nine states there was a modest (though statistically insignificant) increase in unintentional shootings. But a subsequent analysis found that the effect within the felony-prosecution states is largely driven by trends in Florida, which, the authors argue, may be due to several high-profile cases in Florida that enhanced public awareness of the existence of that state's law.[22]

In any case, these findings are at least suggestive that well-publicized laws that encourage gun owners to store their guns safely, and threaten them with criminal sanctions if they do not, may have some effect in reducing unintentional shootings. If a vigorously implemented national policy can reduce unintentional gunshot injuries to children by 41%, the value of these benefits to society will be on the order of $100 to $270 million per year.[23] The costs of this policy are more difficult to quantify. Our lower-bound estimate is that at least 5 million households would be affected by a national safe-storage requirement (that is, have children plus at least one gun stored unsafely).[24] Assuming that these laws do in fact reduce unintentional shootings to children by 41% and have no substantial effect on defensive gun use, a nationwide safe-storage policy makes sense so long as the costs per affected household are no greater than around $20 to $50 per year.

Sentence Add-Ons for Gun Crimes Many states attempt to deter criminals from using guns by threatening a sentence enhancement. A new version of this approach is for state officials to exploit the stiffer sentences available in the federal system, singling out defendants accused of using or carrying a gun for prosecution on federal charges. This approach has been implemented with great fanfare in Richmond, Virginia, as part of "Project Exile," which has served as a model for proposed law-enforcement interventions in other cities as well.[25]

Formal evaluations support the idea that sentencing enhancements can reduce the use of guns in crime, and thereby save lives. Economists Daniel Kessler of Stanford and Steven Levitt of the University of Chicago examined the effects of California's Proposition 8 referendum, which, when adopted in 1982, imposed additional prison terms for repeat offenders convicted of one of several serious felonies (murder, rape, robbery, aggravated assault with a firearm, and burglary).[26] Kessler and Levitt find that the serious felonies that are subject to the new sentence enhancements decreased relative to rates of other crimes in California following Proposition 8, and that this divergence exceeded what was observed for the rest of the United States over the same period. The result is an implied 20% reduction in targeted crimes seven years after the referendum. More directly relevant is an evaluation of sentence-enhancement laws in Florida, Michigan, and Pennsylvania for gun use in felonies, which also found a deterrent effect.[27]

In light of these encouraging results, it is worth considering the costs and benefits of administering a sentence-enhancement provision for gun crimes in the United States as a whole. The benefits of such a program could come at substantial cost. The burden on taxpayers of expanding the prison population (at $40,000 per inmate-year), not to mention the costs to the convicts and their families, are not trivial.[28]

Since we cannot readily quantify the costs of the statewide policies evaluated by Kessler and Levitt and McDowall and colleagues, we instead focus on the costs of implementing the well-documented Project Exile program in Richmond. Criminal-justice records suggest that between February 28, 1997, when Project Exile went into effect, and March 14, 1999, a total of 215 people have been sentenced to prison through the program, with an average sentence of around 4.5 years.[29] Of course some of these people would have been sentenced through state courts in the absence of Project Exile; if we ignore this possibility, then the incarceration costs for project convicts have been on the order of $39 million during this period.

How effective would Project Exile need to be in order to produce benefits that outweighed these costs (ignoring the additional enforcement, prosecution, and publicity expenditures associated with the effort)? Observers from across the spectrum—ranging from the National Rifle Association, to major newspapers such as the *New York Times* and the *Washington Post*, to Virginians Against Handgun Violence[30]—have suggested that Project Exile has been responsible for reductions in gun-assault injuries of about 30% each year since its implementation. These claims surely overstate the program's effects, since gun violence has been decreasing rapidly throughout the United States during the late 1990s and the best bet is that Richmond would have shared in this trend even without the project. If we assume instead that Project Exile reduced gun violence by just 15 to 20%, then the program produced benefits through March 14, 1999, on the order of $150 to $240 million.[31] Even allowing for additional costs of incarceration and the cost of managing and publicizing the program, it appears to be a winner.[32]

Gun Design

Presumably everyone agrees that there should be some limit on the types of weapons that are made accessible to private individuals in America—few of us would sleep better knowing that anyone who passed a standard background check could acquire portable missiles capable of shooting down commercial jetliners or weapons of mass destruction such as nerve gas or atomic bombs. Yet there remains some controversy about where these lines should be drawn and how responsive the design of weapons that are made available should be to consumer-safety concerns.

Bans on Specific Guns Policymakers have implemented bans on particular guns or gun accessories because they are deemed to have design features that increase the lethality of gun misuse, yet are not crucial for sporting uses or self-defense. The ultimate effect of such bans on crime will depend in large part on the degree to which functionally equivalent substitutes are left unaffected by a particular regulation. Federal restrictions on fully automatic machine guns, high-capacity magazines for semiautomatic firearms, and particular types of ammunition (such as armor-piercing handgun ammunition)[33] should effectively raise the price of these technologies to criminals over the long term.[34]

The result is likely to be some reduction in the lethality of gun misuse, though there is admittedly little direct empirical evidence to support our hypothesis.

Similarly, policymakers have long discussed the possibility of banning certain cheap, small handguns commonly referred to as "Saturday Night Specials." If such bans eliminate the manufacture and import of all handguns with design features that are particularly useful for criminal activity—such as short barrels that makes guns easily concealed and carried in public—then criminals will be forced to acquire such guns from the secondary market at a higher price, which in turn should result in some reduction in criminal gun use.[35]

In contrast, the Crime Control Act of 1994 forbids the manufacture and sale of a handful of semiautomatic firearms that were designated as "assault weapons." The guns that were designated as assault weapons were semiautomatic pistols and rifles with military styling, defined as having two or more of the following features—a bayonet lug, flash suppressor, protruding pistol grip, folding stock, or threaded muzzle.[36] Yet aside from aesthetic considerations, in most other respects the banned guns were functionally equivalent to other semiautomatic weapons that were not banned. Because criminals can easily substitute nearly identical weapons for those that have been banned, the net effect on the price of accessing semiautomatic weapons with particular design features is negligible. While it is still too early to draw definitive conclusions about the actual effects of the assault-weapons ban,[37] our expectation is that the long-run effects are likely to be quite modest.

Mandatory Changes in Gun Design The notion that inherently dangerous consumer products can be made at least somewhat safer has been important within the public health community since the time of Ralph Nader's efforts to improve automobile design in the 1960s.[38] Such efforts have been more controversial for firearms—some groups oppose changes to gun design because they infringe on the liberty of gun owners, while others oppose such changes because they don't go far enough to reduce the danger of gun misuse.

Many of the design changes that have been proposed will do little to change the essential features of guns (thereby having only minimal impact on the rights of gun owners), yet may help reduce unintentional shootings. For example, guns can be made inoperable by small children by increasing the pressure that is required to pull the trigger, a design change that should have almost no effect on the ability of adults to operate these weapons. Many unintentional shootings with semiautomatic weapons occur because a bullet is left chambered in the weapon even when the magazine holding the rest of the ammunition is removed from the gun. One study by the Government Accounting Office suggests that devices indicating whether a gun has a round in the chamber (a "loaded-chamber indicator") might prevent up to 23% of unintentional shootings.[39] But too little is known about the situations under which loaded-chamber indicators or related technologies (such as magazine safeties)[40] can prevent unintentional injury or the costs of such devices to facilitate a systematic benefit-cost calculation.

We are also encouraged by the prospect of personalized gun technologies, which prevent guns from being fired by persons other than the authorized owner. This technology holds some promise for saving lives by making guns inoperable to despondent teenagers, curious children, or the criminals who are responsible for around 500,000 gun thefts per year.[41] Some observers are concerned that the introduction of personalized gun technologies may have some offsetting effect on gun violence by increasing overall gun-ownership rates. But in our judgment, if some such safety-conscious people acquire a gun, the potential risk is slight. One of the main advantages of personalized guns is to enhance safety among those people who are not particularly safety conscious.

Currently, 71% of all American adults (and 59% of gun owners) support requirements that all new handguns be sold with personalized gun technology.[42] As of this writing, one manufacturer (Sigarms) was preparing to bring a personalized gun to market that can only be fired after the operator enters a personal identification number into a keypad underneath the barrel, at a cost of about $150 above the price of a similar gun without such a device.[43] Several companies offer devices that retro-fit existing guns to make them operable only by users who wear special magnetic rings, at prices that range from $70 to $300 per gun.[44] Another manufacturer (Colt's) has received a $500,000 grant from the National Institute of Justice to develop a gun that can only be fired when the operator is wearing a special wristband that sends radio signals to the weapon, and the Clinton Administration has asked for $10 million for the 2001 fiscal year budget for the development of such technology.[45] And Oxford Micro Devices is working to develop a handgun that recognizes the owner's fingerprints, which, Oxford estimates, would add only around $100 to the price of the gun once the technology is fully developed.[46] Despite what most people seem to assume, these different technologies need not have equivalent effects on public health. It is true that each of the personalization strategies have the potential to reduce unintentional injuries and suicides and can make guns useless to burglars. But only fingerprint-based technologies have the potential to essentially force all secondary-market transfers to go through a licensed gun dealer, since changing the firearm to respond to a new set of fingerprints will be beyond the technical capabilities of most private citizens.

The net benefit that would be required to make the costs of personalized gun technology outweigh the benefits is quite modest indeed. Suppose, for example, that personalized gun technologies as ultimately developed will add $100 to the purchase price of a new gun. If the only effect of this technology is to prevent one shooting per 10,000 units sold (by making these guns inoperable to thieves), such a policy would pay for itself. Our best guess is that the effects of personalized gun technology should easily clear this bar, given that currently it appears that every 10,000 handguns sold are involved in about 3,000 robberies and assaults and 100 homicides.[47]

Where Next?

We conclude by outlining a policy agenda that, in our judgment, holds considerable promise for reducing the burden of gun violence. First on our list is the regulation of secondary-market gun sales, which is the main source of guns used in crime. The regulation of secondary-market sales could be accomplished, for example, by the mandatory registration of all handguns, a policy that is supported by 82% of all adults and even 72% of gun owners.[48]

While a gun registration plan was proposed as part of the Handgun Control and Violence Prevention Act of 1995,[49] the measure was defeated by those who fear that such a system would make it easier for government to confiscate all guns some day in the future. Yet there exist compromise schemes that would enable law enforcement to regulate secondary-market sales, but preserve the anonymity of gun owners under most conditions. For example, Congress could require that all transactions be channeled through FFLS, and that FFLS report every transaction to ATF (identifying the gun but not the buyer).[50] Such a system would enable ATF to trace crime guns to their current legal owner but, since records are kept by private gun dealers, would not result in a national registry of guns that could be used as part of a gun-confiscation program. A related system would enable gun owners themselves to keep the only records of their transactions, who would then be required to make these records available to law enforcement authorities only in cases where the gun is later used in a crime.[51]

Second, we note that the best available evidence suggests that police patrols against illegal gun carrying may produce benefits far in excess of measurable costs. The question is whether these substantial net gains are outweighed by the intangible costs of such policies, including the resentment that such programs may engender among those who are stopped and searched. While the imposition is primarily on residents of targeted high-crime neighborhoods, the benefit also accrues primarily to these neighborhoods. The expansion of such efforts deserves serious consideration, with particular attention given to the concerns and preferences of the residents of impacted neighborhoods.

Third, we are encouraged by evidence suggesting that sentence enhancements may reduce gun violence. While incarceration imposes considerable costs on society, our calculations suggests that the benefits of sentence add-ons may far outweigh the costs.

We also support the public health community's call to regulate firearms as consumer products. In the case of firearms, many of the costs associated with current gun designs are external to the owner, providing a rationale for regulation that even an economist can appreciate. We also support alternatives to direct regulation that would achieve the same end. For example, a requirement that gun owners purchase insurance for their firearms could substitute the premium-setting process for direct regulation in providing an incentive for enhanced safety features. The most important design change is the development of personalized (or "smart") guns. While a personalized gun would be more expensive, even a small gain in public safety would be sufficient to make it worthwhile.

Our final suggestion is that Congress fund the collection of better scientific data on gunshot injuries, or better yet, on all types of injury.[52] For fatal injuries, we note the Department of Transportation's Fatal Accident Reporting System as a start. For serious nonfatal injuries, an expansion of NEISS may be sufficient. The goal would be to collect detailed information about the circumstances, victim, nature and treatment of injuries, and so forth. Presumably one reason that such a system has not yet been put in place is that it might cost several million dollars per year to develop and administer. Yet given the enormous costs that gun violence impose on society each year, the potential benefits from such data in the form of improving program design and gun policy are considerable.

We have not considered more radical policy shifts such as a national ban on handguns, in part because little is currently known about the net effects of such a change on public safety, or the value of the other intangible costs that such a policy would impose on gun owners. In any event, a handgun ban is infeasible in the current American political context. In contrast, our proposals enjoy broad support and should have little impact on the ability of most people to keep guns at home for protection or sport.[53]

The bottom line is that the current policy regime has left us with a gun problem that imposes substantial costs on everyone in America. Gun violence can be reduced, and many of the interventions designed to separate guns from violence essentially pay for themselves.

Data Sources for Injury and Mortality Rates

In this appendix, we discuss the data sources used to generate the estimates presented in Chapter 2 for the incidence and patterns of fatal and nonfatal gunshot wounds in the United States; as it turns out, information for the former is more reliable and detailed than for the latter. The appendix also includes additional results that expand on those contained in the figures to Chapter 2.

Incidence and Pattern of Fatal Gunshot Wounds

Estimating the number of fatal firearm injuries in the United States each year is fairly straightforward, because law enforcement and public health authorities almost always find out when someone suffers a fatal gunshot wound. The National Center for Health Statistics Vital Statistics program publishes a census of deaths in the United States based on death certificate reports submitted by state agencies. Cause-of-death information comes from the death certificate reports of physicians, medical examiners or coroners, who in almost all states are required to investigate all deaths that result from violence. This information is recorded on death certificates using the *International Classification of Diseases, 9th Revision* (ICD-9), including external cause-of-injury codes (or E codes). Demographic characteristics of the decedent are also recorded on the death certificate by the medical examiner. Additional personal information is typically obtained by the funeral director from informants who are familiar with the decedent. Funeral directors are instructed to gather the information from (in order of preference) spouses, parents, children of the decedent, another relative, or someone else. Since 1989, Vital Statistics mortality files have included information on educational attainment and marital status.

Another source of data on the background characteristics of gunshot victims comes from the 1993 National Mortality Followback Survey (NMFS), which is a nationally representative sample of all deaths to U.S. residents (excluding those from South Dakota) in 1993. For the NMFS study, 22,957 death certificates were drawn from the 1993 Current Mortality Sample, which in turn is a 10% sample of death certificates received by the National Center for Health Statistics from the states. The NMFS oversamples deaths to minorities and youths age 18 to 34 and deaths due to injuries. Data from death certificates were supplemented with information from next-of-kin obtained through telephone or in-person surveys conducted by the U.S. Bureau of the Census. The response rate for the next-of-kin surveys was 83%. Detailed questions were asked about the decedent's employment status, family income, wealth, educational attainment, usual occupation, and health status during the year before death, among other things. Sampling weights are provided with the NMFS to account for the sampling design and non-response.[1]

Mortality rates are defined as the number of people who suffer fatal injuries divided by the number of people in the population. For convenience, these mortality rates are typically scaled up and reported as deaths per 100,000 (rather than deaths per person). In chapter 2 and the tables at the end of this appendix, we calculate mortality rates for different population subgroups defined by gender, age, race/ethnicity, educational attainment, employment, and family income from all sources. The numerators for these rates are calculated from the 1996 Vital Statistics and 1993 NMFS datasets, while the denominators are calculated using data from the Current Population Survey (CPS). The annual CPS is a nationally representative probability sample of the civilian noninstitutional population, conducted by the U.S. Department of Commerce's Bureau of the Census. Each month, roughly 56,000 households are interviewed about employment-related issues. Households are retained in the sample for four months and are then dropped from the sample for eight months, after which they reenter the monthly sample again for four months. We use data from the March CPS interview, also known as the Annual Demographic File, which asks each member of the sampled households detailed questions about educational attainment, work experience, and other socioeconomic characteristics. Population projection weights are provided with the CPS, which adjust for both the sampling design and survey nonresponse.[2]

Incidence of Nonfatal Gunshot Wounds

Estimating the number of nonfatal firearm injuries is more difficult than deriving such figures for fatal gunshot wounds because the former must be pieced together from a number of different sources. Most nationally representative probability samples of American households will contain too few gunshot survivors to support reliable estimates. The best source of data for nonfatal injuries is the National Electronic Injury Surveillance System (NEISS). The NEISS data are derived from a nationally representative probability sample of 91 hospital emergency departments, chosen to support national estimates for consumer-product injuries. NEISS provides information on the discharge status of the ED visit, which allows us to identify those cases that are hospitalized, and also identifies the race, age, and sex of the victim. Sampling weights are provided with the NEISS to facilitate projections to population counts.[3]

Information on cause-of-injury comes from assigned NEISS personnel who are stationed at each hospital and draw information from medical records. The NEISS provides information on injury nature and intent that is similar to what is available with the ICD-9 diagnosis and e-codes, though the NEISS injury information does not use this coding system. Since June 1992, NEISS coders have collected information to identify ED visits due to nonfatal firearm injuries. From June 1992 to September 1992, CDC sponsored a pilot study to determine the proportion of nonfatal firearm injuries identified by NEISS coders. CDC investigators visited a sample of 12 NEISS EDs and independently reviewed ED records and trauma registry listings to compare to the sample of gunshot injuries identified by NEISS coders. The results of this pilot suggested that NEISS coders accurately identified 92% of confirmed gunshot injuries.[4] The NEISS sample has averaged around 3,500 gunshot cases per year.

Since some gunshot victims never seek hospital treatment, estimates derived from the NEISS system will undercount the total number of gunshot injuries. We estimate that for every 100 victims treated in an ED, an additional 19 are treated in a doctor's office and 7 only receive treatment in the field. Both of these estimates are based on rather scant information. We estimate the number of people treated in the doctor's office from the 1995–96 National Ambulatory Medical Care Survey (NAMCS), counting only those doctor's office visits where the victim reports that he was not previously treated in the ED and was not referred by the doctor to the ED. (This estimate is based on just 4 gunshot cases in the pooled NAMCS data.) The other implication of the small sample is that we cannot calculate separate estimates for doctor's office cases by injury intent, even though such cases will presumably consist disproportionately of unintentional injuries that tend to be less severe than suicides and assaults. We estimate the number of people treated at the scene from the 1987–1994 National Crime Victimization Survey (NCVS) data. The NCVS only includes criminal cases, so we are forced to assume that this proportion is similar for suicides and unintentional injuries even though this may not be the case. There are a total of only 64 gunshot injuries (60 treated in the ED and four treated at the scene or at someone's house) in the NCVS. By comparison, May et al. found that 90% of Washington, D.C., inmates who had been shot sought treatment in the ED.[5]

Unfortunately, there is little reliable information available on the socioeconomic characteristics of gunshot survivors, and as a result we are unable to examine the patterns of nonfatal gun violence within the population.

Detailed Injury Results

Tables A1 through A8 supplement the figures reported in Chapter 2 by providing more detailed injury results, including results for more narrowly defined population subgroups. Table A1 shows the trends in intentional, unintentional, and self-inflicted gunshot injuries during the 1993–1997 period broken down by the outcome of the injury (fatality, emergency department treatment, or treatment outside of the ED). These results reveal that there was a proportionally larger reduction in nonfatal than fatal gunshot injuries during the 1990s, which in turn implies either that the proportion of all gunshot injuries that result in a fatality has increased over time, or that there has been some systematic change in the error associated with measuring nonfatal gun injuries. Most of the apparent change in the case-fatality rate seems to have been driven by gun suicides—in 1993 the proportion of gun suicide injuries that were fatal was 70%, while it had increased to 82% by 1997; in contrast, there were only modest increases in the case-fatality rate for gun assaults and unintentional shootings (from 16 to 18%, and 5 to 7%, respectively).

Tables A2 through A7 present detailed firearm mortality rates per 100,000 by injury intent, sex, age, and socioeconomic status. One of the interesting features of these data is that the patterns of inequality in firearm mortality observed among young people ages 18 to 29—rates that are higher for minorities than whites, and higher among the unmarried, those with less schooling, and those who are not employed or with low incomes—are observed among the older cohorts as well. Whatever the mechanisms through which low socioeconomic status elevates the risks of gun violence, they are not limited to the young.

Table A8 provides additional information about the background characteristics of gun suicide victims in the NMFS, in-

Table A1

Incidence of Firearm Injuries in the United States, 1993–97

	Fatal firearm injuries[a]	Nonfatal firearm injuries (ED-treated)[b]	Nonfatal firearm injuries (Non-ED)[c]	Total firearm injuries
1993				
Total	39,595	104,079	27,060	170,735
Self-inflicted	19,213	6,405	1,665	27,283
Assault	18,839	76,422	19,870	115,131
Unintentional	1,543	21,251	5,525	28,319
1994				
Total	38,505	89,703	23,323	151,531
Self-inflicted	19,021	6,270	1,630	26,921
Assault	18,110	68,428	17,791	104,329
Unintentional	1,374	15,005	3,901	20,280
1995				
Total	35,957	84,201	21,892	142,050
Self-inflicted	18,708	5,709	1,630	25,901
Assault	16,010	62,080	17,791	94,231
Unintentional	1,239	16,412	3,901	21,918
1996				
Total	34,040	69,420	18,049	121,509
Self-inflicted	18,389	4,872	1,267	24,528
Assault	14,503	48,335	12,567	75,405
Unintentional	1,148	16,213	4,215	21,576
1997				
Total	32,436	64,207	16,694	113,337
Self-inflicted	17,775	3,018	785	21,578
Assault	13,688	50,980	13,255	77,923
Unintentional	973	10,209	2,654	13,836

Notes:

[a] From the Vital Statistics census of deaths in the United States, taken from the CDC WONDER system. We assme that the distribution of cases where intent is unknown (300 to 400 fatal firearm injuries per year) is similar to the distribution of cases where intent is known.

[b] Estimates from the National Electronic Injury Surveillance System (NEISS).

[c] To account for nonfatal gunshot injuries treated outside of the ED, we estimate the ratio of nonfatal doctor's office- to ED-treated gunshot injuries (0.19) from the 1995–96 National Ambulatory Medical Care Survey and the ratio of untreated to ED-treated gunshot injuries (0.07) from the National Crime Victimization Survey.

Table A2

Firearm Homicide Rates for Males in the United States

	Males 18–29 (rate per 100,000)	Males 30–54 (rate per 100,000)	Males 55 and older (rate per 100,000)
White non-hispanic	5.4	3.9	1.7
Black non-hispanic	133.5	37.6	10.9
Hispanic	38.5	16.4	4.6
Other	10.7	5.5	2.3
Married	12.8	5.4	1.9
Not married	31.4	16.1	5.1
High school dropout	60.0	21.0	3.3
High school degree	37.6	12.8	3.6
At lest some college	6.1	3.4	1.4
Employed	20.6	8.5	4.7
Not employed	51.2	34.7	3.3
Family income			
under $14,000	79.2	41.1	7.4
$14,000–$24,999	38.1	22.1	7.3
$25,000–$49,999	16.2	7.2	2.0
$50,000 or more	4.1	2.1	N/A

Notes: For race, marital status, and educational attainment, the numerators of the mortality rates are calculated using the 1996 Vital Statistics census of deaths, while denominators are calculated using the 1996 Current Population Survey (CPS). For employment status and family income, numerators come from the 1993 National Mortality Followback Survey, while denominators come from the 1993 CPS.

cluding a more detailed breakdown of the health problems for male and female victims. Each of our indicators of poor health in the year before death is subject to some measurement error: victims who have been hospitalized overnight or admitted to a nursing home may have done so for reasons related to the gunshot injury that caused their demise, rather than some preexisting condition; our category of "serious health problems" includes some conditions (such as lung illnesses) that may include relatively mild cases; and some families may have "excessive" medical expenditures in the year prior to the decedent's death

Table A3

Firearm Homicide Rates for Females in the United States

	Females 18–29 (rate per 100,000)	Females 30–54 (rate per 100,000)	Females 55+ (rate per 100,000)
White non-Hispanic	1.6	1.6	0.8
Black non-Hispanic	11.2	6.6	1.8
Hispanic	3.6	2.4	0.7
Other	2.1	1.0	0.3
Married	2.1	1.6	0.9
Not married	3.9	3.6	0.8
High school dropout	6.6	4.5	0.8
High school degree	4.7	3.0	1.0
At least some college	1.5	1.2	0.6
Employed	2.5	2.3	0.9
Not employed	5.8	4.7	1.4
Family income			
under $14,000	11.6	11.8	2.2
$14,000–$24,999	1.1	3.6	0.9
$25,000–$49,999	0.3	2.1	1.4
$50,000 or more	1.3	N/A	N/A

Notes: For race, marital status, and educational attainment, the numerators of the mortality rates are calculated using the 1996 Vital Statistics census of deaths, while denominators are calculated using the 1996 Current Population Survey (CPS). For employment status and family income, numerators come from the 1993 National Mortality Followback Survey, while denominators come from the 1993 CPS.

simply because treatment of the gunshot injury is unusually expensive. Nevertheless, taken together our results suggest that a substantial proportion of gun suicide victims have at least one of these markers (as seen in the last row of Table A8), and that the proportion of gun suicide victims with these markers is higher than what is observed among the victims of motor vehicle crashes (Chapter 2).

Table A4

Firearm Suicide Rates for Males in the United States

	Males 18–29 (rate per 100,000)	Males 30–54 (rate per 100,000)	Males 55+ (rate per 100,000)
White non-Hispanic	16.6	16.0	26.8
Black non-Hispanic	16.5	8.5	11.0
Hispanic	10.4	7.4	9.9
Other	9.2	3.9	3.4
Married	11.8	9.6	17.3
Not married	16.5	22.7	45.9
High school dropout	19.6	17.0	26.4
High school degree	24.3	19.9	29.8
At least some college	7.6	9.3	17.4
Employed	12.3	10.1	12.3
Not employed	17.8	43.6	32.0
Family income			
under $14,000	29.5	38.4	48.8
$14,000–$24,999	20.0	29.3	29.8
$25,000–$49,999	9.5	11.7	21.0
$50,000 or more	4.0	2.1	4.7

Notes: For race, marital status, and educational attainment, the numerators of the mortality rates are calculated using the 1996 Vital Statistics census of deaths, while denominators are calculated using the 1996 Current Population Survey (CPS). For employment status and family income, numerators come from the 1993 National Mortality Followback Survey, while denominators come from the 1993 CPS.

Table A5

Firearm Suicide Rates for Females in the United States

	Females 18–29 (rate per 100,000)	Females 30–54 (rate per 100,000)	Females 55+ (rate per 100,000)
White non-Hispanic	2.2	3.1	2.3
Black non-Hispanic	1.4	1.2	1.1
Hispanic	1.3	1.1	0.5
Other	1.5	1.0	0.6
Married	1.7	2.0	1.8
Not married	2.0	3.8	2.2
High school dropout	2.5	2.7	1.3
High school degree	2.8	3.4	2.6
At least some college	1.2	2.0	1.9
Employed	2.0	1.8	1.5
Not employed	2.5	3.7	2.5
Family income			
under $14,000	3.1	5.4	2.1
$14,000–$24,999	3.3	4.0	2.7
$25,000–$49,999	1.6	2.1	2.8
$50,000 or more	0.9	0.8	1.1

Notes: For race, marital status, and educational attainment, the numerators of the mortality rates are calculated using the 1996 Vital Statistics census of deaths, while denominators are calculated using the 1996 Current Population Survey (CPS). For employment status and family income, numerators come from the 1993 National Mortality Followback Survey, while denominators come from the 1993 CPS.

Table A6

Rates of Fatal Unintentional Shootings for Males in the United States

	Males 18–29 (rate per 100,000)	Males 30–54 (rate per 100,000)	Males 55+ (rate per 100,000)
White non-Hispanic	1.3	0.6	0.7
Black non-Hispanic	3.2	0.9	0.7
Hispanic	1.7	0.4	0.2
Other	1.0	0.2	0.0
Married	0.9	0.5	0.5
Not married	1.8	0.9	0.9
High school dropout	3.1	1.0	0.7
High school degree	2.2	0.9	0.8
At least some college	0.5	0.3	0.4
Employed	2.3	0.6	1.2
Not employed	2.3	2.6	0.7
Family income			
under $14,000	5.7	3.2	1.5
$14,000–$24,999	3.5	1.8	1.8
$25,000–$49,999	1.6	0.4	0.6
$50,000 or more	N/A	N/A	N/A

Notes: For race, marital status, and educational attainment, the numerators of the mortality rates are calculated using the 1996 Vital Statistics census of deaths, while denominators are calculated using the 1996 Current Population Survey (CPS). For employment status and family income, numerators come from the 1993 National Mortality Followback Survey, while denominators come from the 1993 CPS.

Table A7

Rates of Fatal Unintentional Shootings for Females in the United States

	Females 18–29 (rate per 100,000)	Females 30–54 (rate per 100,000)	Females 55+ (rate per 100,000)
White non-Hispanic	0.2	0.1	0.1
Black non-Hispanic	0.2	0.1	0.0
Hispanic	0.1	0.0	0.0
Other	0.0	0.0	0.0
Married	0.2	0.1	0.1
Not married	0.1	0.2	0.1
High school dropout	0.2	0.1	0.1
High school degree	0.3	0.1	0.1
At least some college	0.1	0.1	0.1
Employed	0.2	N/A	0.2
Not employed	0.7	0.1	0.2
Family income			
under $14,000	1.2	0.3	0.5
$14,000–$24,999	N/A	N/A	N/A
$25,000–$49,999	0.2	N/A	N/A
$50,000 or more	N/A	N/A	N/A

Notes: For race, marital status, and educational attainment, the numerators of the mortality rates are calculated using the 1996 Vital Statistics census of deaths, while denominators are calculated using the 1996 Current Population Survey (CPS). For employment status and family income, numerators come from the 1993 National Mortality Followback Survey, while denominators come from the 1993 CPS.

Table A8

Characteristics of Firearm Suicide Victims

	Total (%)	Males (%)	Females (%)
Male	87.0		
Age of death			
15–24	15.9	15.8	17.3
25–34	17.6	17.6	18.5
35–44	16.4	16.4	15.3
45–54	13.3	12.4	19.2
55–64	10.7	9.9	16.1
65–74	13.7	14.5	8.3
75 plus	12.3	13.4	5.3
Indicators of poor health			
1. Victim ever lived in/admitted overnight to nursing home, hospice, or other health care facility	6.1	6.0	7.0
2. Victim had serious health problem[a]	24.0	25.2	15.7
3. Victim homebound last year of life	1.1	1.1	1.5
4. Victim reqd medical assistive device[b]	8.7	9.2	5.6
5. Victim's family had "excessive" medical expenditures year before death[c]	1.1	1.3	0.0
6. Victim had difficulty with household chores year before death[d]	28.6	29.2	24.5
Proportion with chronic illness			
1 & 2	30.3	31.2	24.3
1, 2, & 3	30.4	31.3	24.6
1, 2, 3 & 4	31.7	32.5	26.5
1, 2, 3, 4, & 5	31.9	32.7	26.5
1, 2, 3, 4, 5, & 6	41.5	41.9	39.7

Notes: Estimates obtained from 1,237 gunshot suicide fatalities from the 1993 National Mortality Followback Survey (NMFS), using the NMFS sampling weights to adjust for oversampling.

[a] Defined as those who have suffered a stroke, have Alzheimer's, dementia, senility, or some other organic brain impairment, cancer, or a lung illness (emphysema or bronchitis). We also include cirrhosis cases, though in practice no gunshot suicides had this disease.

[b] Victim required one of the following: infusion pump; shunt, catheter, tube, or surgically inserted access device in vein to allow for infusion of fluids, medication or intravenous feeding while living at home during last year of life; dialysis equipment; or oxygen or devices for breathing therapy.

[c] The NMFS provides information on the family's total out-of-pocket expenditures on medical care for the decedent during the year before death. It is not possible to determine how much of this spending was devoted to treatment for the injury that resulted in death versus other medical care during the year. Further, the NMFS does not identify total medical care spending from all sources. We assume that decedents whose families personally paid more than twice the average medical cost of a fatal gunshot suicide (as reported in Cook et al., 1999) were chronically ill.

[d] Defined as difficulty with the following activities because of physical or mental illness: lifting objects weighing as much as 10 pounds; climbing a flight of stairs; walking a quarter mile; shopping for food; going outside of the home alone; light work around the home; preparing meals; managing money; getting around home; eating; using toilet; bathing/showering; dressing.

Computation of Net Medical Cost Estimates

This appendix provides additional details about the medical-cost calculations presented in Chapter 5. We begin by discussing our methods for estimating the lifetime medical costs for treating gunshot victims. We then review our methods for estimating the lifetime medical costs that gunshot victims *would have* experienced had they *not* been shot.[1]

Costs of Medical Treatment

Our procedure for estimating the costs of medical treatment for gunshot injuries begins with local data from New York and Maryland on hospital acute-care costs, and from South Carolina for acute-care costs for patients who are treated in the emergency department (ED) and released. We rely on state rather than national data to estimate acute-care costs out of necessity. South Carolina is one of the few states to provide data on ED charges, coded by external cause. New York and Maryland are unusual in providing external-cause codes for hospitalized cases and data on costs. Costs and charges are often quite different.[2] (The fact that South Carolina's data are for charges, not costs, is a limitation of our analysis.) Since we intend to project national costs from these local data, we adjust our acute-care estimates for the possibility that these three states may be atypical of the nation as a whole with respect to either the prices of medical inputs (for example, New York may be more expensive than other parts of the country) or types of gun injuries (for example, rural areas like South Carolina may have more unintentional shootings to arms and legs, while urban areas like New York may have more gun assaults or suicides to vital body parts). After making these adjustments, we add on estimates derived from various national data sources to account for follow-up and other medical costs. In what follows, we discuss each step of this method in greater detail.

Method

In our approach, the national medical cost for each category of gunshot injuries is calculated as the product of two estimated magnitudes, the number of gunshot cases and the average cost per case in that category. Table B1 outlines the key data sources that we used to estimate medical costs. Because the available data sources are focused on different levels of treatment, we organize our estimates according to the highest level of medical treatment the patient has received—hospital-admitted, ED only, and "other." This last category includes untreated cases, both fatal and nonfatal, and nonfatal cases treated in doctors' offices. Our estimates start with average acute-care costs; we used data from New York and Maryland for hospitalized cases and from South Carolina for ED-only cases. Lifetime follow-up costs were calculated using a number of national data sources. The lifetime cost per case of each sort was then multiplied by the estimate for the number of gunshot cases of that sort.

Since this method starts with acute-care costs estimated from data in three states, one concern with our procedure is that the acute-care costs of gunshot injuries in these three states may not be representative of those in the nation as a whole. In particular, one source of variation in costs across states may be differences in the injury case mix. In rural states unintentional injuries involving long guns may account for a relatively large share of the case mix (for example, from hunting accidents), while in urban states gun assaults committed by handguns may be relatively more common. In order to control for this potential problem, we use our three-state data to estimate costs for specific types of gunshot injuries. These injury

Table B1

Data Sources for Estimating the Medical Costs of Treating Gunshot Injuries

Type of gunshot injury (highest level of treatment)	Incidence	Acute-care costs	Physician fees	Follow-up medical costs	Payment source
ED-only	1994 NEISS[a]	1997 South Carolina ED discharge data[a]	1992–94 CHAMPUS[b]	1987 NMES[c], 1979–1987 DCI[b]	1992–96 NHAMCS[a], 1997 South Carolina ED[a]
Hospitalized	1994 NEISS[a]	1994–95 Maryland[a] and 1994 N.Y.[a] hospital discharge data	1992–94 CHAMPUS[b]	1987 NMES[c], 1979–1987 DCI[b]	1994 HCUP[a], 1996 NHDS hospital discharge data[a]
Serious disability (spinal cord injuries)	1994 NEISS[a], 1988–1992 NSCISC[a]	1988–92 NSCISC[a]	1988–92 NSCISC[a]	1988–92 NSCISC[a]	1988–92 NSCISC[a]
Death	Vital statistics[a]	1994–95 Maryland HDD[a], 1994 NY HDD[a]	1992–94 CHAMPUS[b]	N/A	1994 HCUP[a], 1997 South Carolina ED[a], 1993 NMFS[a]

Note:

[a] Dataset identifies gunshot injuries using either ICD-9 E-codes or other injury identification system.

[b] Dataset does not provide E-codes or other information to allow us to distinguish between gunshot injuries and non-gun injuries within the same ICD-9 injury diagnosis code.

[c] Dataset includes too few injuries to calculate separate estimates disaggregated by ICD-9 injury diagnosis code. Instead, we estimate the ratio of follow-up medical costs during the first six months to acute-care treatment costs for all injuries, regardless of weapon type or body part injured.

groupings are defined along several dimensions, including (1) injury outcome (fatal/nonfatal), (2) the highest level of medical treatment received (hospitalized, ED-only, or other), (3) victim's sex and age, and (4) diagnosis and external cause-of-injury codes from the *International Classification of Diseases, 9th revision (*ICD-9*)*. The ICD-9 diagnosis codes allowed us to distinguish cases according to body part injured. The ICD-9 external cause-of-injury codes ("E-codes") identify the injury intent (self-inflicted, unintentional, assault), whether the injury was caused by a firearm and, if so, the gun type (handgun, shotgun, rifle).

We multiply our estimates for the average costs per injury type by estimates for the number of gunshot injuries per type (known as the "incidence" of gunshot injuries), calculated from national data. As a result, our method should produce nationally representative cost estimates even if the case mixes in New York, Maryland, and South Carolina are somewhat different from what is observed in other parts of the country.

Incidence As described in Chapter 2, we estimate the incidence of fatal gunshot injuries using data from the Vital Statistics census of deaths, which provides detailed information on the nature of the decedent's injury (in the form of ICD-9 diagnosis codes and E-codes), as well as the victim's sex and age, and whether the victim died as a hospital inpatient, as an ED patient (which under our definition includes dead-on-arrival cases and those for whom hospital-admitted status was unknown), or outside of the ED or hospital (such as dead at the scene). The incidence of nonfatal injuries are estimated using data from the National Electronic Injury Surveillance System (NEISS), a national probability sample of hospital emergency departments.[3] Case studies suggest that NEISS coders record 92%-97% of gunshot injuries treated in sampled EDs.[4] While NEISS uses a system different than the ICD-9 to provide injury characteristics, we use a system that matches NEISS injury codes with ICD-9 diagnosis and E-codes. We adjusted the NEISS estimates for the fact that some gunshot victims receive emergency medical treatment outside of hospital EDs.

Costs for Hospitalized Victims. With slight variations, the life-time cost per hospitalized gunshot survivor was computed using the formulas in equations (B1) and (B2).

(B1) $\text{ShortTerm} = (\text{HospCosts}) \times (1 + \text{FeeRat}) \times (\text{Readmit}) \times (1 + \text{PostDisch})$

(B2) $\text{LC} = (\text{ShortTerm}) \times (\text{LongTerm}) \times (1 + \text{Claims})$

where:

ShortTerm	=	Costs during the first six months following the injury
HospCosts	=	Hospital costs for initial hospitalization
FeeRat	=	Ratio of inpatient professional fees to hospital costs
Readmit	=	Average number of hospital admissions per gunshot injury
PostDisch	=	Ratio of costs in the first six months after discharge to acute inpatient care costs
LC	=	Lifetime medical cost per gunshot survivor
LongTerm	=	Ratio of total lifetime costs to ShortTerm
Claims	=	Ratio of claims administration costs to total lifetime medical costs

Hospital costs for gunshot injuries are based on a census of hospital discharges in Maryland in 1994–1995 (2,852 cases) and New York in 1994 (3,835 cases). Around 7% of victims in each state were deceased at discharge. We focused on hospital discharge data (HDD) from Maryland and New York because these states require that hospitals provide E-codes for all injury-related hospital discharges. More importantly, regulatory agencies in these states ascertained costs of care by hospital service, and as a result the charges reported in these hospital-discharge datasets can be converted to reasonably accurate estimates of actual hospital costs.

The ratio of professional fees to hospital costs (*FeeRat*) was calculated at the diagnosis-code level using the 1992–1994 Civilian Health and Medical Program of the Uniformed Services (CHAMPUS) data, which are based on payments (including co-pay) in an insured population of 2 million military dependents and non-Medicare retirees.[5] While CHAMPUS is the best available data source for estimating professional fees, the lack of E-codes meant that we had to calculate professional-fee ratios by diagnosis without regard to whether the injury was by gunshot or other means.

The ratio of ancillary and follow-up costs in the first six months to all acute inpatient care costs (*PostDisch*) was calculated from the 1987 National Medical Expenditure Survey (NMES).[6] These follow-up costs include emergency transport, prescriptions, medical supplies (such as crutches), home health care, and follow-up doctor's visits (but not follow-up hospitalizations). Because NMES contains only 397 total hospital-admitted injuries, we could not produce estimates for *PostDisch* that are specific to individual ICD-9 diagnosis- or E-codes. Instead, we used NMES to estimate that *PostDisch* is equal to 11.8% for *all* injuries, regardless of the body part injured or method of injury.

Some gunshot victims will have repeat hospitalizations in the short term that are not captured by *PostDisch*. To adjust for this fact, we used Missouri hospital-discharge data from 1994 that include individual patient-identification numbers to estimate the average number of hospital admissions that each gunshot victim has during the first year following the injury (*Readmit*). We multiplied the Maryland/New York estimates of costs per *admission* by our Missouri estimate of total first-year hospital admissions per victim to obtain an estimate of hospital costs per gunshot *case*.

Except for catastrophic spinal cord injuries (SCI) and traumatic brain injuries (TBI), we estimated long-term follow-up medical costs by calculating for each ICD-9 diagnosis code the fraction of lifetime medical payments for treating an injury that is incurred during the first six months, and then converting it to a ratio (*LongTerm*). Our estimate for *LongTerm* comes from the National Council on Compensation Insurance's Detailed Claims Information (DCI) dataset, which provides a sample of 452,000 injury cases (including 138,000 hospitalized cases) that occurred from 1979 through 1987.[7] The advantage of the DCI dataset is that it is one of the few sources of lifetime medical costs. The disadvantages of the DCI are that it provides information only at the diagnosis- but not E-code level, only includes injuries that occur at work, is somewhat dated, and in some states excludes injuries that involve less than 3 to 9 days of work loss.

As an example of how these components combine to form average costs per case, consider an unintentional gunshot injury to the abdomen with initial hospitalization costs (*HospCosts*) equal to $10,000 and professional payments equal to 30% of the hospitalization costs (*FeeRat* = 0.3). Suppose that on average patients with such injuries are hospitalized 1.1 times during the first year (*Readmit* = 1.1), that other follow-up costs during the first 6 months equal 70% of hospitalization costs (*PostDisch* = 0.7), and that the DCI data suggest that lifetime medical costs for injuries within this ICD-9 diagnosis code are twice the total costs incurred during the first six months (*LongTerm* = 2.0). Lifetime costs then equal ($10,000 $\times$ 1.3 $\times$ 1.1 $\times$ 1.7 $\times$ 2.0) = $48,620.

The calculation is slightly different for TBIS, for which we made some additional adjustment for lifetime custodial-care costs that are unlikely to be fully captured by the *LongTerm* factor. The Bureau of the Census reports an annual cost of $84,285 (inflated from 1993 to 1994 dollars using the CPI-All Items) for custodial care in a public mental-retardation facility.[8] We followed previous studies[9] in assuming that TBI care in an intensive care facility costs twice the Census Bureau's custodial-care figure.

We produced separate estimates for the lifetime medical costs for SCIS because these relatively rare catastrophic cases account for a disproportionately large share of the overall costs of treating gun injuries. We estimate lifetime medical charges using data from the National Spinal Cord Injury Statistical Center (NSCISC) on 820 gunshot-related SCIS treated between 1988 and 1992 in 24 model spinal-cord injury-treatment centers.[10] We converted estimates for inpatient hospital charges into costs using Medicare cost-to-charge ratios for the SCI hospitals.

Finally, we controlled for the possibility that Maryland and New York medical prices may not be nationally representative by deflating our cost estimates using the Health Care Finance Association's Hospital Wage Index values for October 1, 1994.[11]

This hospital wage index should closely approximate overall variation in medical costs in light of a recent case study suggesting that 80% of total hospital operating expenses come from employee costs.[12] We also multiply lifetime medical costs by 1.03 or 1.04 (depending on the patient's primary payment source) to reflect claims administration costs.[13]

As seen in Table B2, we estimate that the average costs for acute-care treatment of nonfatal, hospitalized gunshot injuries

Table B2

Medical Costs per Case for Nonfatal Hospitalized Gunshot Injuries: Hospital Discharge Data for Maryland, 1994–95, and New York, 1995

Injury intent	N	Acute-care costs	Hospital readmits	6 month ancillary & follow-up costs[a]	Post-6-month follow-up costs[b]	Claims ad-min. costs[c]	Total lifet. co
Maryland 1994–95							
All GSW	2,394	$16,932	$680	$2,081	$19,907	$2,294	$42,
Unintentional	516	$13,651	$579	$1,681	$12,400	$1,666	$29,
Self-inflicted	50	$33,985	$1,051	$4,140	$12,118	$3,276	$54,
Assault	1,470	$18,078	$734	$2,223	$23,927	$2,626	$47,
Intent unknown	357	$14,554	$555	$1,785	$15,301	$1,691	$33,
New York 1994							
All GSW	3,334	$16,634	$616	$2,038	$18,006	$2,200	$39,
Unintentional	600	$15,011	$575	$1,842	$23,560	$2,528	$43,
Self-inflicted	69	$35,932	$776	$4,337	$44,609	$6,055	$91,
Assault	2,503	$16,770	$631	$2,056	$16,111	$2,033	$37,
Intent unknown	163	$12,411	$446	$1,519	$15,499	$1,925	$31,

Notes: Figures are in 1998 dollars. Lifetime medical costs calculated using a 3% real discount rate
[a] Estimate is an average across all injuries of follow-up costs during first six months, calculated from the 1987 NMES data.
[b] Follow-up costs beyond the first six months are estimated at the diagnosis-code level from the DC worker's compensation data.
[c] Claims administration costs are calculated separately by the patient's expected payer. Estimated ratios for injuries are 0.03 (all gunshots), 0.04 (unintentional), 0.03 (self-inflicted), and 0.03 (assaults)
[d] Note that total cost column may not equal sum of other columns; total costs are calculated by first multiplying together the lifetime cost factors for each case and then calculating the average of this product, which may not equal the product of the averages.

in Maryland and New York are remarkably similar ($16,932 versus $16,634 in 1998 dollars), as are the total lifetime costs ($42,092 versus $39,494). In both Maryland and New York, nonfatal self-inflicted gunshot injuries have higher lifetime costs than unintentional injuries or assaults.

The medical costs of fatal hospital-admitted gunshot injuries ($15,135 in Maryland and $14,694 in New York) are on average less than half those for nonfatal cases (Table B3). The difference between fatal and nonfatal hospital-admitted gunshot cases highlights the magnitude of follow-up treatment costs. For the nonfatal gunshot injuries shown in Table B2, the majority of medical treatment costs come after the patient has been discharged from the hospital (54% in Maryland and 58% in New York).

Costs for Emergency-Department-Only Injuries We estimated medical charges for gunshot survivors admitted to the emergency department but not admitted to the hospital using a census of ED discharges from South Carolina for 1997. The South Carolina dataset provides information on 796 ED-only gunshot injuries, and includes those who were dead on arrival to the emergency room. While these data are not from our reference year (1994), and they have charge rather than cost data, they are the best available data on this subject. We estimated follow-up medical costs using the ancillary and follow-up factors described in equations (B1) and (B2) above.

As seen in Table B4, the lifetime charges associated with ED-only gunshot injuries in South Carolina average $1,516 for non-fatal cases and $2,747 for fatal cases.

Costs for Non-ED Cases No dataset provides reliable information on nonfatal gunshot injuries each year in which the victim does not seek medical treatment at the ED or hospital. Since these cases are likely to account for only a very small share of total costs, we ignore them in our cost calculations. For fatal non-ED gunshot injuries (cases where the victim dies on the spot), we assumed that the medical costs equal the cost of emer-

Table B3

Medical Costs per Case for Fatal Hospitalized Gunshot Injuries: Hospital Discharge Data for Maryland, 1994–95, and New York, 1995

Injury intent	N	Acute-care costs	Ancillary costs[a]	Claims admin. costs[c]	Total lifetime cost[d]
Maryland 1994–95					
All GSW	200	$13,077	$1,485	$575	$15,135
Unintentional	21	$10,426	$1,171	$568	$12,166
Self-inflicted	37	$10,204	$1,145	$406	$11,755
Assault	107	$15,289	$1,746	$646	$17,681
Intent unknown	35	$11,413	$1,228	$535	$12,659
New York 1994					
All GSW	258	$12,564	$1,424	$705	$14,694
Unintentional	29	$15,812	$1,808	$996	$18,617
Self-inflicted	26	$9,021	$1,006	$334	$10,361
Assault	188	$12,997	$1,470	$723	$15,142
Intent unknown	15	$7,465	$822	$554	$8,842

Notes: Figures are in 1998 dollars. Lifetime medical costs calculated using a 3% real discount rate. Accute care estimnates include $443 per case for coroner costs.

[a] Estimate is an average across all injuries of follow-up costs during first six months, calculated from the 1987 NMES data.

[b] Follow-up costs beyond the first six months are estimated at the diagnosis-code level from the DCI worker's compensation data.

[c] Claims administration costs are calculated separately by the patient's expected payer. Estimated ratios for injuries are 0.03 (all gunshots), 0.04 (unintentional), 0.03 (self-inflicted), and 0.03 (assaults).

[d] Note that total cost column may not equal sum of other columns; total costs are calculated by first multiplying together the lifetime cost factors for each case and then calculating the average of this product, which may not equal the product of the averages.

gency transport to the medical examiner, equal to $193,[14] plus the costs of the coroner's examination, equal to $487.[15]

Payment Sources We estimate the payment sources for hospital-admitted gunshot injuries using data from the Agency for Health Care Policy and Research's Healthcare Cost and Utiliza-

Medical Costs per Case for Emergency-Department (ED)-Only Gunshot Cases

jury tent	Cases (N)	ED charges	6 mo. follow-up doctor/clinic visits[a]	6 mo. ancillary & follow-up costs[a]	Post-6-month follow-up costs[b]	Claims admin. costs[c]	Total lifetime costs[d]
onfatal 1997 South Carolina ED data							
ll gunshot	796	$1,049	$228	$39	$153	$45	$1,516
nintentional	351	$1,003	$216	$37	$107	$45	$1,408
lf-inflicted	22	$2,175	$249	$38	$294	$69	$2,824
ssault	342	$1,059	$236	$41	$140	$38	$1,515
tent unknown	89	$902	$250	$36	$377	$64	$1,629
tal 1997 South Carolina ED data							
ll gunshot	41	$2,244	0	$410	0	$93	$2,747

tes: Figures are in 1998 dollars. Sample includes both fatal and nonfatal injuries.

stimate is an average across all injures of follow-up costs during first six months, calculated from the 87 NMES data.

ollow-up costs beyond the first six months are estimated at the diagnosis-code level from the DCI worker's mpensation data. We estimate the percent of total medical costs incurred during the first six months om the DCI data for each diagnosis code, and then multiply one minus this proportion by the sum of e ED charges and other medical costs incurred during the first six months. Our estimates for the pro-rtion of medical costs incurred during the first six months after the injury are 0.92 (all gunshot wounds), 3 (accidents), 0.90 (self-inflicted), and 0.91 (assault).

laims administration costs are calculated separately by the patient's expected payer. Estimated ratios r injuries are 0.03 (all gunshots), 0.04 (accidents), 0.03 (self-inflicted), and 0.03 (assaults).

Jote that total cost column may not equal sum of other columns; total costs are calculated by first ltiplying together the lifetime cost factors for each case and then calculating average of this product, hich may not equal the product of the averages.

tion Project (HCUP) for 1994, which includes an E-coded sample of hospital discharges from California, Connecticut, Massachusetts, Maryland, New Jersey, New York, Washington, and Wisconsin. For nonfatal cases, we also used the 226 gunshot cases from the National Hospital Discharge Survey (NHDS) for 1996, a nationally representative sample of discharges from 500 hospitals with 63% of cases E-coded. For fatal hospitalized injuries, we replicated the HCUP estimates using the National Mortality

Followback Survey (NMFS), a nationally representative sample of U.S. decedents in 1993 that includes 2,764 gunshot victims. Estimated payment sources for ED-only gunshot injuries come from the 1997 ED discharge data from South Carolina. We also estimated the distribution of primary payers for ED-only cases using pooled data from the 1992–96 National Hospital Ambulatory Medical Care Survey (NHAMCS). The NHAMCS provides information on primary payment source, but not on total costs or charges. The five years of pooled NHAMCS data contain 129 gunshot cases.

Table B5 presents our estimates for the primary source of payment for gunshot victims according to the patient's highest level of treatment and injury outcome (fatal/nonfatal). These primary payers apparently bear most of the medical costs for gunshot injuries, with secondary and third payers bearing relatively little of the total cost. In the bottom panel of Table B5, we present descriptive information from several of our datasets on the proportion of patients who receive *any* payments from the specified source. We see, for example, that the proportion of acute-care patients who have private or commercial insurance as their first source of payment (30%) is quite close to the proportion of such patients who have insurance as any one of their top five sources of payment (32%). Since this is true for most of the payment sources across the three datasets for which we have information on multiple payers, we may conclude that most gunshot victims have only one source of payment.

Limitations

Our estimates for the costs of treating gunshot injuries substantially improve the quality of information that is available about these costs. Nevertheless, these findings are subject to several qualifications stemming from limitations with the available data. Our estimates for the national costs of hospital treatment come from data from only two states. Unfortunately, no other states both require hospitals to E-code discharge records and provide information that can identify actual medical costs. Our estimates for follow-up medical costs come from NMES and

Table B5

Payment Sources for Gunshot Injuries by Level of Treatment/Nature of Injury

	ED-only		Hospital admitted survivors		Disabled survivors—spinal cord injuries 1988–92 (N=820)		Fatal cases		
	NHAMCS 1992–1996 (N=129)	SC 1997 (N=796)	HCUP 1994 (N=4404)	NHDS 1996 (N=226)	Acute care	5 yrs. Post-discharge	Hospitalized 1994 (N=370)	ED-only 1997 (N=41)	All 1993 (N=2764)
Primary Payer									
Priv/comm insurance	18.8%	25.6%	21.9%	22.1%	30.0%	11.5%	18.7%	34.1%	24.7%
Medicaid	17.2	8.9	35.5	29.1	55.1	54.2	32.2	2.1	11.2
Worker's comp	2.3	0.9	1.5	2.0	2.1	4.2	0.6	0.0	1.1
Medicare	1.5	4.2	2.0	2.2	2.0	28.1	5.7	4.9	11.3
Other government	0.0	1.0	9.5	5.9	3.3	2.1	6.4	0.0	5.3
No payer (indigent)	0.8	0.8	0.1	1.6	6.0	0.0	0.0	0.0	23.5
Self pay	52.7	56.8	26.9	27.4	1.3	0.0	33.1	53.7	21.3
Other	6.5	1.9	2.6	9.7	0.7	0.0	3.4	4.9	1.4
All sources of payment									
Priv/comm insurance	Not available	Not available	Not available	Not available	31.7%	17.7%	Not available	Not available	37.6%
Medicaid					61.0	64.6			13.4
Worker's comp					2.4	4.2			3.0

Table B5 (*Continued*)

	ED-only		Hospital admitted survivors		Disabled survivors—spinal cord injuries 1988–92 (N=820)		Fatal cases		
	NHAMCS 1992–1996 (N=129)	SC 1997 (N=796)	HCUP 1994 (N=4404)	NHDS 1996 (N=226)	Acute care	5 yrs. Post-discharge	Hospitalized 1994 (N=370)	ED-only 1997 (N=41)	All 1993 (N=2764)
Medicare					2.5	32.3			16.0
Other government					7.8	5.2			8.3
No payer (indigent)					6.1	0.0			22.8
Self pay					1.3	0.0			47.3
Other					1.2	1.0			2.2

Notes: Spinal cord injury estimates come from model system data from the National Spinal Cord Injury Statistical Center database; acute-care data are available for 820 patients who suffered injuries between 1986 and 1992, for whom five-year follow-up data are available for 96 cases (see text). Distributions for all sources of payment (where available) may sum to more than 100 since some patients have multiple sources of payment. Hospitalized fatal case estimates come from the 8-state 1994 HCUP-3 hospital discharge dataset (CA, CT, MA, MD, NJ, NY, WA, and WI).

DCI data that do not allow us to specifically identify costs for gunshots distinct from other types of injuries. The DCI data are further restricted to workplace injuries. Finally, our E-coded ED discharge data from South Carolina provide information on charges, not costs.

Potentially the most important limitation with our estimates for treating gunshot injuries concerns cases resulting in permanent disability, which account for a large share of total medical costs. While we developed separate estimates for one type of catastrophic case that may result from gunshots—spinal cord injuries—there are other types of costly disabilities that may also be caused by gunshot injuries. We estimated the lifetime medical costs for these other injuries using somewhat dated NMES and DCI data that did not allow us to distinguish gunshots from other injuries within the same ICD-9 diagnosis code. Our estimates will understate the actual lifetime costs of treating gunshot injuries if gunshots are more likely than other injuries with the same diagnosis to result in long-term disability. Our attempts to develop separate lifetime cost estimates for other types of disabilities were hampered by limited charge, payment, or cost information for long-term care from available data sources. Improving surveillance and cost data for gunshots resulting in long-term disability is the highest priority in any effort to further refine the estimates presented here.

Counterfactual Medical Costs

As discussed in Chapter 5, our estimates for the medical costs that would-be gunshot victims *would have* incurred had they *not* been shot rest crucially on our assumptions about what the victim's life expectancy and medical expenses would have been, as well as how workers who suffer fatal gunshot injuries are replaced in the local economy and the extent to which there is weapon substitution. In order to examine the sensitivity of our estimates to these assumptions, we develop estimates under different assumptions regarding two of the most important unknowns—the nature of worker replacement, and weapon substitution.

We consider two different possibilities regarding worker replacement. In the first scenario, all workers who suffer fatal gunshot injuries are replaced by immigration into the local economy. In this case, under the *status quo* a hypothetical victim suffers a fatal gunshot injury and society's medical expenditures equal the costs of treating the wound, plus whatever medical treatment the replacement worker receives over the course of her lifetime (Table B6). Under the counterfactual scenario of no gun violence, society would have incurred only the lifetime

Table B6

Net Medical Costs from Fatal Gunshot Injuries to Employed Victims under Different Assumptions about Worker Replacement

	Status quo (with gunshot injuries)	Counterfactual (no gunshot injuries)	Difference (net costs to medical system)
Worker replacement through immigration			
Fatal gunshot injuries	Treatment costs for gunshot injury	LME of would-be victim	Treatment costs for gunshot injury
	Lifetime medical expenses (LME) of replacement worker		
Worker replacement from unemployed population			
Fatal gunshot injuries	Treatment costs for gunshot injury	LME of would-be victim	Treatment costs of gunshot injury
	LME of replacement worker	LME of would-be replacement worker	minus
			LME of would-be victim

Notes: We assume that for nonfatal gunshot injuries, total lifetime medical costs equal the costs of treating the gunshot injury, plus the victim's regular lifetime medical expenses (LME).

medical expenses of the would-be victim; thus, the change in medical expenditures caused by the gunshot injury equals the costs of treating the victim. However, Table B6 shows that when workers are replaced by unemployed residents of the local economy, under the counterfactual scenario of no gun violence, society incurs lifetime medical expenses for both the would-be victim *and* her replacement; as a result, the net change in medical spending caused by a fatal gunshot injury in this case equals the costs of treating the injury less the lifetime medical expenses of the would-be victim.

Our assumptions about weapon substitution differ for gun assaults, suicides, and unintentional shootings, and as a result we discuss our assumptions for each injury intent in turn.

Assaults

What happens to medical expenditures when gun assaults are eliminated? The answer depends in large part on what happens to the behavior of perpetrators once guns are no longer available. Previous research suggests that gun availability affects the lethality but not the level of violent crime.[16] As a result, we assume that under some intervention that eliminates the use of guns in assault, perpetrators substitute other weapons for guns to commit their assaults. Since knives are the most lethal likely substitute for guns in violent assault, we conservatively assume that each gun assault is replaced by a knife assault. The substitution of knives for guns thus changes the level of medical spending by affecting the mix of crimes in three ways:

1. First, some of those who would have died as a result of gunshot injuries now suffer fatal knife injuries instead. Since the fatality rate for knife assaults is one-third that of gun assaults,[17] the number of cases in this category equals one-third the number of gun homicides. For these cases, the net costs of gunshot injuries to the medical system are given by the average costs of treating a fatal gunshot injury times the number of fatal gunshot injuries, minus the costs of treating a fatal knife injury times the number of fatal gunshot injuries. Most studies assume that the costs of treating a fatal injury are the same regardless

of the weapon that is used,[18] which we follow in our own calculations. Thus, the net medical costs of these cases equals zero.

2. Second, some of those who would have suffered fatal gunshot injuries now suffer nonfatal knife wounds. The number of such cases equals two-thirds the number of fatal firearm assaults, by the logic given above. If we assume that workers are replaced by immigrants, then the net costs of these cases equal the average costs of providing medical treatment for a fatal gunshot injury ($Costs_{GSW}$) times the number of gunshot wounds (N_{GSW}), minus the costs of providing treatment to a nonfatal knife wounds ($Costs_{KW} \times N_{GSW}$), as in equation (3). We must also subtract the average lifetime medical expenses (LME) for victims who are not working $(1 - P_{work}) \times (N_{GWS})$, since the elimination of gun violence creates a partially offsetting increase in medical expenses for treating these survivors.[19] We do not subtract out the lifetime medical costs for workers, since they are replaced by immigrants under our maintained assumptions.

(B3) Net costs $|_{Immigration} = (Costs_{GSW} \times N_{GSW}) - (Costs_{KW} \times N_{GWS}) - (LME) \times (1 - P_{work}) \times (N_{GSW})$

If, on the other hand, workers who suffer fatal gunshot injuries are replaced by unemployed current residents of the society, then we must net out LME for all gunshot victims, as in equation (B4).

(B4) Net costs $|_{Local\ Replacement} = (Costs_{GSW} \times N_{GSW}) - (Costs_{KW} \times N_{GSW}) - (LME) \times (N_{GSW})$

3. Finally, those who would have suffered nondisabling, nonfatal gunshot injuries now suffer nondisabling, nonfatal knife wounds. The net medical costs from these cases equal the difference in costs of treating nonfatal gun versus knife wounds.

Tables B7 and B8 present our estimates for the gross, counterfactual, and net medical costs for all gun assaults in 1997; estimates expressed on a per-injury basis can be obtained by dividing these figures by the number assaults in 1997 reported in the left-hand column. The two tables differ in that the former

Table B7

Net Medical Costs of Gunshot Injuries in 1997, Assuming Complete Worker Replacement through Immigration

	Costs of treating gunshot injuries	Counterfactual medical costs	Net costs
Assaults (1997 cases = 77,923)	$1.436	$0.553	$0.883
Unintentional shootings (1997 cases=13,836)	$0.309	$0.012	$0.297
Suicides (1997 cases=21,578)			
Perfect weapon substitution	$0.116	$0.116	$0
No weapon substitution	$0.116	$0.308	−$0.192
Weapon substition only for chronically ill victims	$0.116	$0.199	−$0.083
All gunshot injuries (1997 cases=113,337)			
Upperbound	$1.862	$0.682	$1.180
Lowerbound	$1.862	$0.873	$0.989

Notes: See Appendix B for additional details about calculations. Figures in billions.

assumes that employed victims of fatal gunshot injuries are replaced in their jobs through immigration, while the latter table assumes replacement from local unemployment rolls. The important point is that both tables suggest that the net medical costs for gun assaults are far lower than the gross costs of treating gunshot victims for their injuries.

Unintentional Gunshot Injuries

Logic dictates that when unintentional shootings are averted through some public policy measure, there should be no off-

Table B8

Net Medical Costs of Gunshot Injuries in 1997, Assuming Complete Worker Replacement through Unemployed Residents of Local Area

	Costs of treating gunshot injuries	Counterfactual medical costs	Net costs
Assaults (1997 cases = 77,923)	$1.436	$0.756	$0.680
Unintentional shootings (1997 cases=13,836)	$0.309	$0.032	$0.277
Suicides (1997 cases=21,578)			
Perfect weapon substitution	$0.116	$0.116	$0
No weapon substitution	$0.116	$0.641	−$0.525
Weapon substition only for chronically ill victims	$0.116	$0.401	−$0.285
All gunshot injuries (1997 cases=113,337)			
Upperbound	$1.862	$0.905	$0.957
Lowerbound	$1.862	$1.430	$0.432

Notes: See Appendix B for additional details about calculations. Figures in billions.

setting increase in knife or other accidents. As a result, eliminating unintentional shootings produces net savings to the medical care system in two ways:

1. Those who would have suffered fatal unintentional gunshot injuries are now able to live the rest of their lives. If we assume that victims would have been replaced by immigrants, the net savings equal the average costs of treating a fatal unintentional shooting times the number of injuries minus the average lifetime medical costs of victims times the number of would-be victims times the proportion who are not working, as in equation (B5).[20]

(B5) Net costs $|_{\text{Immigration}} = (\text{Costs}_{\text{GSW}} \times N_{\text{GSW}}) - (\text{LME}) \times (1 - P_{\text{work}}) \times (N_{\text{GSW}})$

If we instead assume that victims would have been replaced by local residents who had previously not been working, the net costs are given as in equation (B6).

(B6) Net costs $|_{\text{Local Replacement}} = (\text{Costs}_{\text{GSW}} \times N_{\text{GSW}}) - (\text{LME}) \times (N_{\text{GSW}})$

2. Those who would have suffered nonfatal gunshot injuries are also spared. Since we assume that the lifetime medical costs of those who suffer nonfatal injuries equal the costs of treating the injury plus the regular medical expenses that the victim would have incurred over the rest of his lifetime, the net savings to the medical-care system from eliminating nonfatal unintentional shootings equals the medical costs of treating these gunshot injuries.

Tables B6 and B7 show that the net medical costs of unintentional shootings range from \$277 to \$297 million.

Gun Suicides

Determining the net medical costs of gun suicides is complicated, since the available research is not clear on how weapon availability influences the number or lethality of suicide attempts. Given this uncertainty, we calculate medical costs for suicide victims under three plausible assumptions about the counterfactual scenario where guns are eliminated from use in suicide attempts. As we will show, depending on our assumptions about weapon-substitution, the net costs of gun suicides to the medical system may be zero or even negative (i.e., savings).

Scenario 1 One possibility is to assume perfect weapon substitution in the case of gun suicides. In the extreme case where weapon substitution is perfect for all suicide attempts, there will be no change in injury outcomes when suicidal individuals substitute other weapons for firearms. The result is that eliminating the use of guns in suicide attempts produces no change in medical expenditures.

Scenario 2 At the other end of the spectrum, we may assume no weapon substitution in suicide attempts. In this case, the net savings to the medical care system are as follows:

1. Those who would have suffered fatal self-inflicted gunshot injuries are now uninjured. The net costs to the medical care system equal the costs of providing medical treatment for the gunshot suicides minus the lifetime medical costs of victims who are not working (equation B7) if we assume workers are replaced by immigrants,[21] or by the lifetime medical costs society would have paid for all victims if workers are instead replaced by unemployed locals (equation B8). We assume that every suicide attempt by chronically ill individuals are "in earnest," and thus the 30 to 40% of attempters who are ill at the time of their attempt fall in this group.

$$\text{(B7) Net costs}\,\big|_{\text{Immigration}} = (\text{Costs}_{\text{GSW}} \times N_{\text{GSW}}) - (\text{LME}) \times (1 - P_{\text{work}}) \times (N_{\text{GSW}})$$
$$\text{(B8) Net costs}\,\big|_{\text{Local Replacement}} = (\text{Costs}_{\text{GSW}} \times N_{\text{GSW}}) - (\text{LME}) \times (N_{\text{GSW}})$$

2. Those who would have suffered nonfatal self-inflicted injuries are now also spared. The net costs to the medical care system equal the costs of providing medical treatment for the gunshot injury.

The net medical costs of treating gun suicides under these assumptions about weapon substitution are given in Tables B7 and B8. While the costs of treating gunshot injuries for those who attempt suicide was around $116 million, the net effect on the medical care system if there is no weapon substitution is to actually reduce overall medical spending by between $192 and $525 million. The reason is that the large majority of gun suicide attempts are almost instantly fatal and thus require little medical treatment, while many of the victims would have had substantial medical bills over their remaining lifetimes.

Scenario 3 Reality is likely to be somewhere between the extreme assumptions underlying scenarios 1 and 2. In practice, some suicide attempts are the result of impulsive behavior, and efforts to keep guns away from such individuals will prevent their suicide attempts altogether. Other suicidal individuals will be more determined (for example, those who suffer chronic or terminal illnesses) and will complete their suicide attempts with some other method that is as dangerous as firearms. Our "intermediate weapon-substitution" scenario assumes that there is perfect weapon substitution for the 40% of cases where the attempter may have a chronic illness, and assumes no weapon substitution for the remaining cases. Thus, the net changes to the medical care system are as follows:

1. The estimated 40% of chronically ill suicide attempters suffer fatal self-inflicted injuries even if guns are unavailable, resulting in no net change in costs to the medical care system.

2. Others who would have suffered fatal self-inflicted gunshot injuries if guns are available now do not attempt suicide through other means. The net change to the medical budget from these cases equals the foregone cost of treating the fatal gunshot injuries and lifetime medical costs for unemployed victims (equation B7) if we assume workers are replaced by immigrants. If we assume workers are replaced by unemployed locals, net medical costs equal the costs of treating gunshot injuries less the lifetime medical costs of all would-be victims (equation B8).

3. Finally, those who would have suffered nonfatal self-inflicted gunshot injuries are spared. The net medical costs equal the costs of providing treatment for these injuries.

The estimated net medical costs under these assumptions about weapon-substitution range from −$83 million to −$285 million (Tables B7 and B8); that is, suicides reduce the nation's medical bill by $83 to $285 million.

Payers

Earlier, we presented estimates of who pays for the medical treatment of gunshot injuries. Yet there is no reason to believe that the sources of payment for the would-be victim's medical expenses had he not been shot would be the same as those responsible for the costs of treating his gunshot injury. For example, many gun homicide victims are young and unemployed, and thus either the hospital or a government health program covers the cost of treating these gunshot injuries. If these victims had not been shot, many would have gone on to join the workforce, in which case future medical expenses would be covered by private health insurance.

To learn more about who would have paid for people's lifetime medical expenses had they not been shot, we use data from the 1998 Current Population Survey (CPS) analyzed by Paul Fronstin of the Employee Benefits Research Institute.[22] These data suggest that 71% of nonelderly Americans (under 65) had private health insurance in 1997, while 15% relied on government programs, and 14% had no health insurance.[23] Among the elderly, fully 96% are covered by Medicare. Table B9 presents our detailed estimates for the net medical costs of gun violence

Table B9

Net Medical Costs of Gunshot Injuries in 1997 Borne by Different Payment Sources

	Net costs to government	Net costs to private insurance	Net costs paid by other sources
Assaults (1997 cases=77,923)			
Worker replacement through immigration	$0.491	$0.155	$0.237
Worker replacement through unemployed local residents	$0.390	$0.073	$0.217
Unintentional shootings (1997 cases=13,836)			
Worker replacement through immigration	$0.142	$0.057	$0.098

	Net costs to government	Net costs to private insurance	Net costs paid by other sources
Worker replacement through unemployed local residents	$0.131	$0.050	$0.096
Suicides (1997 cases = 21,578)			
Perfect weapon substitution			
Worker replacement through immigration	$0	$0	$0
Worker replacement through unemployed local residents	$0	$0	$0
No weapon substitution			
Worker replacement through immigration	−$0.188	−$0.012	$0.008
Worker replacement through unemployed local residents	−$0.444	−$0.068	−$0.013
Weapon substitution only for chronically ill victims			
Worker replacement through immigration	−$0.078	−$0.015	$0.010
Worker replacement through unemployed local residents	−$0.208	−$0.071	−$0.006
All gunshot injuries (1997 cases = 113,337)			
Upperbound	$0.633	$0.213	$0.335
Lowerbound	$0.077	$0.055	$0.300

Notes: See Appendix B for additional details about calculations. Figures in billions.

to different payers under alternative assumptions about worker replacement and weapon substitution.

Limitations

The most important limitation of our analysis is the sensitivity of our estimates to assumptions about worker replacement and, in the case of gun suicides, weapon substitution. We also assume that gunshot victims have life expectancies and annual medical expenses equal to the average expenses of members of the general population of the same sex and age, though in fact gunshot victims may be atypical in both respects. Unfortunately, very little systematic information is available on any of these points, and a comprehensive analysis of these parameters is beyond the scope of the current project.

Computation of Productivity Losses

This appendix discusses our estimation procedure for the lost earnings and household production of gunshot victims. We then present more detailed calculations for lost production and our new cost-of-illness estimates than those contained in the figures for Chapter 6.

Lost Earnings

Our baseline estimates for the lost lifetime earnings of gunshot victims (presented in the first column of Table C1) essentially replicate the methods used in previous studies such as those by Rice, MacKenzie and Associates, Max and Rice, and Miller and Cohen.[1] We first use cross-sectional data from the 1993 Current Population Survey (Appendix A) to estimate the lifetime earnings for men and women in different five-year age groups, assuming a 3% real discount rate. These calculations assume that a 30-year-old man in 1996 would have the same annual earnings at age 60 as a 60-year-old man in 1996; while this approach is standard practice, the resultant estimates are subject to some error because they may confound "age" and "cohort" effects.

Following previous studies, we initially assume that each decedent in the 1996 Vital Statistics data would have had the same lifetime earnings as the average earnings estimated for their sex/age group from the CPS data, and then calculate the average lifetime earnings of victims of gun homicides, suicides, and unintentional shootings. These estimates account for dif-

Table C1
Lost Lifetime Production (Earnings Plus Household Production)

	Traditional COI approach[a]	Modified approach (1)[b]	Modified approach (2)[c]
Decedent's foregone lifetime earnings assumed to equal lifetime earnings of members of the general population controlling for:	sex and age	sex, age, race, and educational attainment	sex, age, race, educational attainment, and initial earnings differences between victim and members of general population
Gun homicide			
Men	$973,626	$557,038	$490,193
Women	$555,383	$464,613	$427,444
Total	$904,564	$542,065	$480,045
Gun suicide			
Men	$684,216	$591,786	$491,182
Women	$482,321	$449,108	$336,831
Total	$650,124	$573,808	$471,529
Unintentional shootings			
Men	$880,974	$605,977	$442,363
Women	$536,219	$284,288	$295,660
Total	$841,100	$595,976	$424,879
All gunshot injuries			
Men	$809,366	$577,948	$489,383
Women	$518,919	$461,083	$378,122
Total	$767,667	$561,119	$473,684

Notes:

[a] We estimate lifetime earnings for different sex and age groups using data from the 1996 Current Population Survey (CPS) March Demographic File, using a 3% real discount rate and assuming th gunshot victims ould have had the same life expectancy as others of the same sex and age. respondents with no income during the year are assigned incomes of zero and retained in the analy sample. To these earnings estimates, we add estimates for household production for men and wom taken from Expectancy Data (1999). We then estimate average lost productivity by weighting

ferences across sex/age groups in life expectancy (and thus years of productivity) and participation in the labor market (by including people in each sex/age group outside of the labor market in calculating average earnings over the life course).

We then make two adjustments to these standard cost-of-illness estimates. First, instead of assuming that gunshot victims would have had the same earnings as people in the general population controlling for sex and age, we assume that victims would have had the same earnings as other people of the same sex, age *and* race and educational attainment. Our second adjustment is to the usual life expectancy assumptions underlying the standard estimates. Previous studies assume that gunshot victims would have the same life expectancy (and thus the same number of productive years) as other people in the general population of the same sex and age. While no dataset is detailed enough to allow us to definitively estimate how long gunshot victims would have lived had they not been shot, using life expectancy figures that are specific to race and educational attainment as well as sex and age is a partial adjustment, since these background characteristics are correlated with health outcomes.[2] These estimates are presented in the second column of Table C1.

Finally, we make another adjustment for the differences in earnings between people in the general population and gunshot victims in the year before their deaths by multiplying the estimates presented in the second column of Table C1 by the earnings ratios presented in Figure 6.4.

ther the earnings for different sex/age groups by the demographic distribution of gunshot victims in e 1996 Vital Statistics census of deaths.

We adjust the first-column estimates by first calculating survival probability figures that are ecific to sex, age, race and educational attainment. We also calculate lost earnings for different x, age, race and education groups from the 1996 CPS and then calculate the averages for gunshot ctims using the average sociodemographic characteristics of victims taken from the 1996 Vital atistics.

n the third column, we multiply the second column estimates by the income ratios presented in gure 6.1.

Table C2

Traditional and Modified Cost-of-Illness (coi) Estimates for Gun Violence in 1997

	Traditional coi[a]	Traditional coi, using better data[b]
Gun assaults (77,923 in 1997)		
Medical	$ 1.436	$ 1.436
Lost production	$13.848	$ 8.293
Total	$15.284	$ 9.729
Gun suicides (21,578 in 1997)		
Medical	$ 0.116	$ 0.116
Lost production	$11.620	$10.244
Total	$11.736	$10.360
Unintentional gunshot injuries (13,836 in 1997)		
Medical	$ 0.309	$ 0.309
Lost production	$ 1.263	$ 0.895
Total	$ 1.572	$ 1.204
All gunshot injuries (113,337 in 1997)		
Medical	$ 1.862	$ 1.862
Lost production	$26.635	$19.456
Total	$28.497	$221.318

Notes: All estimates are in billions of 1998 dollars.

[a] For the traditional coi figure, medical costs equal the estimated costs of treating gunshot injuries in 1997 (presented in Chapter 5). Productivity losses are calculated under the assumption that had they not been shot, gunshot victims would have had the same lifetime earnings as people in the general population of the same sex and age.

[b] For the traditional coi using better data, we assume that gunshot victims would have had the same lifetime earnings and life expectancy as people in the general population of the same sex, age, race, and educational attainment.

New Cost of Illness Estimates

Table C2 presents more detailed information about the new cost-of-illness estimates that underlie Figure 6.6. The table demonstrates that the changes in our cost-of-illness estimates are driven by modifications to estimates for lost productivity and particularly by modifications motivated by conceptual concerns with the cost-of-illness approach. Using better data to estimate what gunshot victims would have earned had they not been shot reduces our overall estimate by around $7 billion.

*Computations of Contingent-Valuation
and Quality-of-Life Estimates*

The first two sections of this appendix provide additional details about the contingent-valuation analysis presented in Chapter 8. Section 1 discusses the econometric model used to conduct the parametric maximum-likelihood analysis, while Section 2 discusses the basis for our estimates of the effects of household characteristics on the probability of supporting the hypothetical violence-reduction program. The third section presents alternative estimates for what the American public would pay to eliminate gun violence based on values taken from studies of wage premiums for risky work and from jury awards in personal injury cases.

Contingent-Valuation Estimates:
Econometric Approach

Our empirical strategy is based on the framework outlined by economists Trudy Cameron and Michelle James.[1] Let Y_i equal the (unobserved) WTP value that respondent (i) has in mind when answering the first and second referendum questions in the NGPS. The respondent will answer in the affirmative to the first referendum question ($I_{1i} = 1$) if the "price" of the program in the form of higher taxes (t_{1i}) is not greater than the respondent's WTP ($Y_i \geq t_{1i}$). Similarly, the respondent will support the program in the follow-up CV question ($I_{2i} = 1$) if the new price t_{2i} is less than WTP ($Y_i \geq t_{2i}$), where t_{2i} is equal to double t_{1i} if I_{1i}

= 1 and half of t_{1i} if $I_{1i} = 0$. We initially assume that Y_i is log-normally distributed (equation E1), which constrains WTP to be positive.

(E1) $\log Y_i = \beta + u_i \qquad u_i \sim f(0, \sigma^2)$

From this setup we can estimate household WTP using the "interval-data" or "double-bounded" model developed by economists Michael Hanemann, John Loomis, and Barbara Kanninen.[2] The probabilities for the four possible joint outcomes for the first (I_{1i}) and second (I_{2i}) referendum questions are given in equations (E2) through (E5) where F represents some cumulative distribute function. (Recall that with the NGPS data, $t_{2i} = 2t_{1i}$ if $I_{1i} = 1$, and $t_{2i} = 0.5t_{1i}$ if $I_{1i} = 0$).

(E2) $P[I_{1i} = 1, I_{2i} = 1]$
$= P[Y_i \geq t_{2i} > t_{1i}]$
$= P[Y_i \geq t_{2i}]$
$= P[u_{1i}/\sigma \geq (\log t_{2i} - \beta)/\sigma]$
$= 1 - F[(\log t_{2i} - \beta)/\sigma]$

(E3) $P[I_{1i} = 0, I_{2i} = 0]$
$= P[Y_i < t_{2i} < t_{1i}]$
$= P[Y_i < t_{2i}]$
$= P[u_{1i}/\sigma < (\log t_{2i} - \beta)/\sigma]$
$= F[(\log t_{2i} - \beta)/\sigma]$

(E4) $P[I_{1i} = 1, I_{2i} = 0]$
$= P[t_{1i} \leq Y_i < t_{2i}]$
$= P[Y_i < t_{2i}] - P[Y_i < t_{1i}]$
$= F[(\log t_{2i} - \beta)/\sigma] -$
$F[(\log t_{1i} - \beta)/\sigma]$

(E5) $P[I_{1i} = 0, I_{2i} = 1]$
$= P[t_{2i} \leq Y_i < t_{1i}]$
$= P[Y_i < t_{1i}] - P[Y_i > t_{2i}]$
$= F[(\log t_{1i} - \beta)/\sigma] -$
$F[(\log t_{2i} - \beta)/\sigma]$

We obtain estimates for the parameters of this model by applying maximum-likelihood estimation (MLE) to the log-likelihood function in equation (E6).

(E6)   In L = $\sum_i$ $(I_{1i})(I_{2i})\{1 - F[(\log t_{2i} - \beta)/\sigma]\} +$
$(1 - I_{1i})(1 - I_{2i})\{F[(\log t_{2i} - \beta)/\sigma]\} +$
$(I_{1i})(1 - I_{2i})\{F[(\log t_{2i} - \beta)/\sigma] -$
$F[(\log t_{1i} - \beta)/\sigma]\} +$
$(1 - I_{1i})(I_{2i})\{F[(\log t_{1i} - \beta)/\sigma] -$
$F[(\log t_{2i} - \beta)/\sigma]\}$

The coefficient estimate for the variables $\log t_{1i}$ and $\log t_{2i}$ is an estimate for $1/\sigma$, which in turn allows us to identify an estimate b for the parameter β. Calculating the standard errors for mean and median household WTP is complicated by the fact that our estimate for b is really the ratio of two estimates—the estimated value for β/σ divided by an estimate for $1/\sigma$. The usual standard error formula for a linear predictor evaluated at some value of the regressors x_0 is given by equation (E7).

(E7) $SE(x_0'b) = (x_0 V x_0')^{1/2}$

In the model without covariates, estimation of the formula in equation (E7) is simplified somewhat because b is a scalar rather than a vector, so V is also a scalar equal to the variance of b, $x_0 = 1$, and (E7) simplifies to (E8).

(E8) $SE(b) = (V)^{1/2}$

The complication in our case comes from the fact that b is actually the ratio of two estimates b'/s', where b' is an estimate for (β/σ) and s' is an estimate for $(1/\sigma)$. In this case the variance for b = b'/s' can be approximated by the formula given in equation (E9).[3]

(E9) $V = Var(b) = Var(b'/s') \approx (b'/s')^2[(Var[b'])/(b')^2 + (Var[s'])/(s')^2]$

The final complication is that (E9) gives us the variance for the estimated mean of the natural log of Y (WTP), while ultimately we are interested in the variance of the predicted mean of the untransformed WTP. With $E[\ln Y] = b$ and $Var(E[\ln Y]) = V$ then the variance of E[Y] is given by equation (E10).[4]

(E10) $\mathrm{Var}(\mathrm{E}[\mathrm{Y}]) = \exp(2b + V)^*(e^v - 1)$

With a point estimate and standard error for b in hand, we can calculate societal WTP. If w_1 represents the NGPS sampling weight for household (i), which equals the number of households in the population that each sampled household represents, then estimated societal WTP is given by equation (E11). While b provides an unbiased estimate for the expected value of log WTP, for a log-normal variable the mean of WTP itself will be given by $\exp(b) \times \exp(0.5\sigma^2)$.[5]

(E11) Societal WTP $= \sum_i w_i \times \exp(b) \times \exp(0.5\sigma^2)$

Detailed Results of the Parametric Analysis

The main findings from the parametric maximum-likelihood analysis are presented in Chapter 8 and suggest that the average household in America is willing to pay on the order of $200 per year to reduce the use of guns in assault by 30%.

In addition to these main results, the effects of the different covariates on household WTP are also of some interest, since these coefficient estimates provide information relevant to both the credibility of the CV responses and the distributional effects of programs to reduce or eliminate gun violence. The effects of the household-level covariates included in our maximum-likelihood model are shown in Table D1. The numbers reported in the table represent the difference in the probability of a supportive vote for the group indicated in the left column versus the comparison group. The presence of children within the home increase the WTP of respondents to reduce gun violence; either respondents are willing to pay more to enhance their personal safety when they have children, or they are reporting on household rather than individual WTP, or both. Finally, respondents in households with guns are less likely to support programs to reduce gun violence.

Table D1

Coefficient Estimates from MLE Estimates, from NGPS Contingent Valuation Referendum Data

Variable	Effect of household background variable on probability of voting "yes" to support program to reduce gun violence by 30%
Race	
African-American	−0.02
Hispanic	−0.05
Other race	−0.08
(White is comparison group)	
Region	
Northeast	0.02
Midwest	−0.06
West	−0.06
(South is comparison group)	
Household composition	
Number of children under age six	0.09**
Number of children between ages 6 and 17	0.04**
Number of adults	−0.01
Family income	
$20–39,999	0.08*
$40–59,999	0.17**
$60,000 plus	0.17**
Income missing	0.03
(Less than $20,000 is comparison group)	
Gun in home	−0.08**
N	1,110
Log likelihood	−759.3

Notes: Figures are in 1998 dollars. Author calculations from applying maximum likelihood estimation to equation (3) for the 1997 gun survey data and equation (11) for the 1998 gun survey data, under the assumption that WTP is normally distributed.

** Statistically significant at the 5% level.
* Statistically significant at the 10% level.

Sensitivity Analysis for the Parametric Analysis

In our baseline parametric analysis, we use household-level covariates because we interpret the CV responses as reflections of household (rather than individual) WTP. If different individuals within the home would report different WTP values, then our estimates should still be unbiased (since adults are randomly selected from households) but may be inefficient. To explore this possibility, we reestimated our preferred MLE model after restricting the sample to married respondents and including an indicator for the respondent's gender. While the coefficient estimate for an indicator variable for husbands is negative and statistically significant, inclusion of this variable serves to reduce estimated mean WTP by less than 7%.

We also find that our estimates are fairly robust to assumptions about the distribution of WTP. Reestimating equation (E6) above (with covariates) under the assumption that WTP has a log-logistic (rather than log-normal) distribution produces an estimated mean WTP of $206. Using a normal distribution, which allows WTP to be negative, produces an estimate of $213.

One concern with these CV data is the possibility that responses to the follow-up CV question are influenced by the initial question. As Cameron and Quiggin note, respondents may become more certain about their response to the second rather than first question because they have had more time to reflect on the public good in question.[6] Alternatively, respondents may believe that the first question provides information about the actual average cost of the public good and may then react negatively to the second question that asks the respondent to pay "more than it costs." The descriptive statistics presented in Table 8.1 provides some evidence to support this second effect. For example, Table 8.1 shows that 69% of respondents who are asked about a $100 tax increase in the first question will pay this much to support the program, though only 51% of those who are asked about a $50 increase in the first question will support a $100 tax increase (76% × 67%).

To address the possibility that the respondent is sensitized by the first CV question, and thus that the first and second questions produce observations from slightly different WTP distributions, we follow Cameron and Quiggin and reestimate WTP using a bivariate probit model. The bivariate probit model allows for different means for the first and second WTP values ($\beta_1 \neq \beta_2$), as well as separate error processes that have different variances ($\sigma_1^2 \neq \sigma_2^2$) and are only imperfectly correlated ($\text{Corr}[u_{1i}, u_{2i}] = \rho < 1$).[7] While the bivariate probit model affords greater flexibility than the MLE model given by equation (E6), this strategy comes at the cost of less precise estimates[8] and makes interpretation of the results somewhat complicated. Our bivariate probit estimates suggest a mean WTP of $309 for the first referendum question and $209 for the second. If responses to the first CV question are more accurate, then the estimates presented in Chapter 8 may somewhat understate societal WTP.

Another concern that commonly arises with CV studies is that of "protest zeroes," defined as cases in which the respondent rejects the hypothetical market scenario even though her true WTP exceeds the stated "price" of the referendum.[9] The proper definition of protest zeroes is complicated in our application. Fairly uncontroversial is the case of tax protestors—those respondents who object to financing the program out of tax revenues, but who would be willing to pay the stated amount to achieve a 30% reduction in gun violence if the program were financed by some other means. One possibility is to identify as tax protesters the 24% of respondents who "strongly agree" with the survey question that "taxes are too high." When we reestimate our model without these respondents in the sample—which is the preferred method for dealing with protesters[10]—our estimate is only 13% higher than the preferred estimate of $239 reported in Chapter 8.

More complicated are cases where the respondent objects to the mechanism for reducing gun violence, rather than the mechanism for financing the program. The NGPS asks about programs that target the illegal use or transmission of firearms, which in turn should reduce gun violence holding the overall crime rate constant. Respondents who object to these interventions should *only* be counted as protest zeroes if alternative interventions exist that could plausibly reduce gun crime without reducing the overall crime rate, which is a debatable proposition. In any case, we classify as intervention-protesters those who "strongly disagree" that "the government should do everything it can to keep handguns out of the hands of criminals, even if it means that it will be harder for law-abiding citizens to purchase handguns." Excluding these respondents produces only a 7% increase in WTP compared with the $239 figure from Chapter 8.

The Quality-of-Life Approach

Previous studies attempt to approximate what the public would pay to reduce gun violence by importing estimates for the value per statistical life or injury from generic studies of marketplace behavior, or from jury awards.[11] This approach has become increasingly common in the health-economics literature. We use this approach to value unintentional shootings and gun suicides, since our contingent-valuation survey provides no information on gun injuries that do not result from an assault. We also estimate the value of reducing gun assault as a basis for comparison with our contingent-valuation-survey results.

We begin by discussing some of the complications that arise from trying to infer what people would pay to reduce gun violence from other studies of the value of life saving and workplace safety.

Nonrepresentativeness of Gunshot Victims

Studies of marketplace behaviors rely on samples of people who may have different attitudes toward risk than those who are at high risk for gunshot injury. For example, estimates for wage-risk tradeoffs are typically derived using samples of workers in their late 30s or early 40s. In contrast, most victims of gun homicide are quite young, while victims of gun suicide are frequently quite old (Chapter 2). If WTP to reduce the risk of death is inversely related to one's age, as many economists assume, then wage-risk studies may overstate the value of one statistical life to those at highest risk for gun suicide and understate the value for those at greatest risk of gun homicide.

One solution to this problem is to convert estimates for the value of one statistical *life* into estimates for the value of one statistical *life-year*.[12] The best available evidence suggests an estimate of $70,000 to $175,000 per year of life,[13] with $100,000 taken to be a reasonable mid-point.[14] What remains somewhat controversial is whether the life years that are saved by public policy interventions should be "discounted" to account for when the life saving occurs. Almost all economists agree that a program that costs $10,000 today and produces $10,000 in cash benefits ten years from now is not a good investment, since the $10,000 could instead be placed in an interest-bearing account that would yield some greater amount in the future. The same logic leads most economists to discount the dollar value of any future health benefits that are achieved by government interventions. Yet not everyone agrees with this logic. Some observers are (rightly) concerned that discounting the value of lives saved off into the future favors those who are currently alive at the expense of future generations—benefits to people's health or the environment that occur 100 or 1,000 years from now will receive very little weight in an evaluation that discounts future benefits at some nonzero rate.[15] A compromise solution is to discount health benefits experienced in future years by people who are currently alive and avoid discounting when the health benefits of programs accrue to future generations.[16]

Yet even if we adjust for age, victims of gun violence are still not representative of the population of workers who are used to estimate these value-of-life figures. An alternative to using the average value for average workers is to use values estimated from more comparable populations. The adjustments could be of two forms. First, the observation that some gun-assault victims have chosen very risky occupations (for example, drug dealing) suggests that they place a relatively low value on their lives. Several studies have found that workers in high-risk occupations are a self-selected group who require relatively small compensation for those risks. A review by Harvard economist Kip Viscusi shows that while the willingness-to-pay to avoid one statistical death among average workers ranges from $3.75 to $8.75 million, estimates derived from workers in high-risk jobs suggest a value-of-life on the order of $1 to $1.5 million.[17] Such people are also more likely than others to smoke or drive unbuckled, further evidence that they place a relatively low value on their lives.[18] If those who are at high risk for gunshot injury are more like workers in risky occupations than average workers, then by their own preferences a lower-than-average valuation is appropriate. Thus, one adjustment that we can make is to multiply estimates for the value of one statistical life by the ratio of the value to workers in risky jobs to the value for the average worker ($1.5 \div 3.75 = 0.4$).

Whether this first adjustment is appropriate for the case of suicides is not clear. Determining what people who are at high risk for suicide—that is, at high risk of intentionally shooting themselves—would pay to reduce the risk that they are shot raises complicated questions about what we mean by people's preferences, and which preferences should be taken seriously. Someone who shoots himself essentially reveals that at the moment that the trigger is pulled, he is willing to pay zero (or even some negative amount) to avoid being shot. Yet many survivors do not attempt suicide again,[19] suggesting that there may be a certain element of impulsiveness and regret associated with at least some suicide attempts. People who suffer from some mental or physical illness that puts them at high risk for gun suicide may be willing to pay some amount to reduce the chance that they will be able to act on such an impulse in the future. It is in this sense that it is meaningful to talk about people's willingness-to-pay to reduce their risk of gun suicide and to compare this payment amount with the compensation required by workers in jobs with higher risks.[20]

Another possibility is to also adjust for income. By one estimate, the value that individuals place on their own lives increases by about 10% for every 10% increase in their income.[21] Given the income differences in average income between gunshot victims and other people documented in Chapter 2, the value of risk-reductions to those at high risk of gunshot injury may be as much as 37% lower than for the general population. Thus we might further adjust our estimates by multiplying by $(1 - 0.37 = 0.64)$. Because workers in risky jobs may also have below-average incomes, adjusting for *both* preferences and income may lead us to understate the value of health and safety to those at high risk of gunshot injury.

Some analysts have argued that the government should use a uniform standard across population groups in regulating risk, without regard to income or preferences of the individuals involved. Risk regulation can then serve as a form of implicit income redistribution, giving the poor more safety than they would be willing to pay for (if given the choice of more safety versus more of other things). Our own preference is to value the benefits of public programs as the beneficiaries actually value them and handle income redistribution separately, rather than hiding implicit choices about redistribution within the details of cost-benefit analysis.

Weapon Substitution

Studies of marketplace behavior estimate the wage that people would require to take a different job with a slightly higher risk of injury or illness but all else held constant. Because these studies assume that all else is equal between the two jobs, the issue of offsetting increases in risks from other workplace hazards is not an issue. Yet a central theme from Chapter 3 is that any consideration of the costs of gun violence must take the possibility of weapon substitution seriously. If some criminal assailants or suicidal individuals substitute other weapons for guns, then any reductions in gun injuries that are achieved may be offset in part or whole by some increase in the number of nongun injuries. Because of the possibility of weapon substitution and the replacement of gun injuries with nongun injuries, what workers will pay to reduce the risk of a fatal workplace accident by 1/10,000 may be different from what people will pay to fund a program that reduces their risk of gunshot injury by 1/10,000. To account for the possibility of weapon substitution, our quality-of-life estimates include some adjustment for the offsetting disutility that people receive from an increase in nongun injuries.

In sum, extrapolating the value of reducing or eliminating the value of gun violence from data on workplace behaviors or jury awards is subject to a number of errors and requires a number of assumptions that may or may not hold. Yet in the absence of contingent-valuation survey data on what the public would pay to reduce rates of unintentional shootings and gun suicide, the quality-of-life approach is our only hope for placing a value on changes in such injuries. Developing estimates along these lines is the subject of the next section.

Quality of Life Estimates

Extrapolating from previous studies of the value of life suggests that the value of eliminating gun violence in America in 1997 is in the range of $20 to $50 billion, equal to between $170,000 and $400,000 per gunshot injury. Different assumptions yield higher and lower estimates, as shown in Table D2. In our judgment, the estimates presented in the third and fourth columns are the most appropriate though, as noted above, even these estimates are likely to be incomplete given that wage-risk studies are likely to ignore many of the benefits to society from reducing or eliminating gun violence.

The first column of Table D2 contains estimates that are similar in spirit to those presented by economists Ted Miller and Mark Cohen, who have developed the only previous WTP estimates for the value of eliminating gun violence.[22] As with the Miller and Cohen calculations, those presented in column one of our table ignore the possibility of weapon substitution. Unlike the Cohen and Miller study, these initial estimates do not discount the value of health benefits that occur in the future (in order to highlight the effects of discounting for those who disagree with this adjustment).

The estimate for fatal gunshot injuries comes from multiplying an estimate for how long the average victim of a gun homicide, suicide, and unintentional shooting would have lived had

imates for What the American Public Would Pay to Eliminate Gun Violence in
)7, Calculated Using the Quality-of-Life Approach

	Baseline, ignore weapon substitution (1)	Baseline, account for weapon substitution (2)	Adjust (2) by discounting future health outcomes using 3% Rate (3)	Adjust (3) for risk aversion of gunshot victims (4)	Adjust (4) for income of victims (5)
saults (=77,923)	$62.3 billion	$35.1 billion	$23.8 billion	$9.5 billion	$6.1 billion
lf-inflicted (=21,578)					
High		$46.7 billion	$33.4 billion	$13.4 billion	$8.6 billion
Low		$0.0 billion	$0.0 billion	$0.0 billion	$0.0 billion
Middle	$46.7 billion	$27.9 billion	$20.0 billion	$8.0 billion	$5.1 billion
nintentional (=13,836)	$5.7 billion	$5.7 billion	$4.4 billion	$1.8 billion	$1.1 billion
l gunshot juries (=113,337)					
High		$87.5 billion	$61.5 billion	$24.6 billion	$15.7 billion
Low		$40.8 billion	$28.2 billion	$11.3 billion	$7.2 billion
Middle	$114.7 billion	$68.7 billion	$48.2 billion	$19.3 billion	$12.3 billion

tes: Figures in 1998 dollars.

he not been shot (equal to 37.4, 25.9, and 35.6 years, respectively), by the value of one year of life estimated from wage-
risk tradeoffs in the labor market ($100,000, as noted above),
times the number of fatal gunshot injuries in 1997. To this
amount we then add the number of nonfatal gunshot injuries
times the value of a nonfatal gunshot injury, which Miller and
Cohen estimate to equal $170,000 using data from jury awards.[23]
Our life expectancy figures are estimated by using data from
the 1996 Current Population Survey and Vital Statistics census
of deaths to calculate the mortality rates for men and women
in different five-year age groups. With these five-year mortality

rates in hand, we estimate the expected life expectancy of people in different sex/age groups, assign each gunshot victim in the Vital Statistics dataset the life expectancy of the average person in the victim's sex / age, and then calculate the average life expectancy for victims in each of the injury-intent groups (homicide, suicide, and unintentional injury).

In principle, one could adjust the assumed life expectancies underlying these estimates to control for the fact that gunshot victims have other sociodemographic characteristics that contribute to shorter life spans than those of other people of the same sex and age. But this raises a number of difficult issues: If what people are willing to pay for a reduction in the risk of death is related to life expectancy, how are expectations of remaining life expectancy formed? Do individuals form these expectations by examining mortality patterns among people of the same sex and age, or is the relevant comparison group defined more narrowly with respect to other sociodemographic characteristics? Are these expectations rational (that is, equal to actual life expectancies on average)? Almost nothing is known on these points, and as a result our default is to use the more simple life expectancy estimates. Using this approach, our calculations suggest that the value of eliminating gun violence in 1997 is on the order of $115 billion, or around $1 million per gunshot injury.

Accounting for the possibility of weapon substitution reduces the estimate to between $41 and $88 billion, with a mid-range estimate of nearly $70 billion (column 2 of Table D2). The additional uncertainty with these modified estimates stems from uncertainty about what would happen to the number of suicides in an environment in which guns are not readily available for misuse.

When we make the additional adjustment of discounting the value of future health benefits using a 3% discount rate (column 3), our estimates are on the order of around $50 billion. (These estimates will be subject to a slight error because for computational simplicity we discount the lifetime gains in health for the average gunshot victim, rather than calculate the average of the discounted gains in health for all gunshot victims). Adjusting for potential differences in risk aversion between gunshot victims and the populations used to estimate the value of a statistical life in previous studies shifts these estimates downward to around $20 billion.[24] We prefer these estimates, which suggest a value per gunshot injury of between $170,000 and $430,000, because they account for the opportunity cost of investing funds in public programs that produce benefits off into the future. Whether the higher or lower of these numbers should be preferred is not clear.

While these estimates are likely to be incomplete (Chapter 4) and rest on a number of assumptions and extrapolations (above), they nevertheless suggest that the benefits of reducing gunshot injuries are far greater than simply the direct, tangible costs from medical spending and lost productivity considered in Chapters 5 and 6.

Notes

Chapter 1

1. *New York Times* (1999).
2. Cannon et al. (1999).
3. Brooke (1999a).
4. Brooke (1999b).
5. Brooke (1999a, p. A1).
6. Ibid.
7. Sink (1999, p. A18).
8. Welsh (1999, p. 28).
9. Firestone (1999, p. A1).
10. Ibid.
11. Ibid.
12. Morrow (1999, p. A1).
13. Spitzer (1998).
14. Clotfelter and Hahn (1978).
15. Viscusi (1993).
16. Anderson (1999).
17. Zimring and Hawkins (1997).
18. Cook and Ludwig (1996).
19. Wilson (1995), p. 494–495.

Chapter 2

1. Ikeda, Gorwitz, James, Powell, and Mercy (1997).
2. Bonnie, Fulco, and Liverman (1999).
3. These are what is known as "crude" death rates. When homicide trends are measured by "age adjusted" death rates (standardized to a particular age distribution of the population), the all-time peak homicide rate occurred in 1974 (Ikeda et al., 1997).
4. Cook and Laub (1998); Blumstein (1995); Fox (1996).
5. Blumstein (1995); Cork (1999); Grogger and Willis (1998).

6. Ikeda et al. (1997).

7. We confirmed this result by performing an analysis of variance on mortality rates defined for all possible groups defined by age, race, high school status, and marital status. The black-white gap shrinks by just 7%, and the Hispanic-white gap by 36%.

8. Kennedy, Piehl, and Braga (1996).

9. See McGonigal et al. (1993) and Schwab et al. (1999).

10. McLaughlin et al. (1998).

11. Peak rates of suicide differ by race and gender: for white men, suicide rates peak in old age and for white women in midlife; for non-white men and women, the peak rates are in early adulthood (see Moscicki, 1995).

12. See Miller and Hemenway (1999) for an excellent review of overall suicide patterns.

13. Miller and Hemenway (1999).

14. Jamison (1999, p. 100).

15. We count as "seriously ill" all gun-suicide victims who had suffered a stroke at some point before their suicide attempt, or had Alzheimer's disease, dementia, senility, or some other organic brain impairment, cancer, or a lung illness (emphysema or bronchitis). We also counted cirrhosis in this group, though in practice no gun-suicide victims had this disease. While on average those citizens with one of the diseases described here will probably be chronically ill, there may be some proportion of cases where the prior or current illness has only modest effects on the person's health.

16. These figures are for 1996, taken from the Centers for Disease Control, National Center for Injury Prevention and Control (CDC, 1996a).

17. Ibid.

18. Authors' calculations using data from the 1996 Vital Statistics Census of Death to estimate the denominator of this rate and data from the 1996 Current Population Survey March Demographic File to estimate the numerator. See Appendix A for additional details about both datasets.

19. Figures originally reported in the *International Journal of Epidemiology*, 27 (1998): 216 downloaded from www.guncite.com on January 24, 2000 (GunCite, 2000).

Chapter 3

1. Montgomery (1980).

2. Sager and Wadler (1980).

3. Miller (1999).

4. See Levitt (1996) and Levitt (1997).

5. Donohue and Siegleman (1998).

6. Ludwig, Duncan, and Hirschfield (2001).

7. Leitzel (1998).

8. Cook and Blose (1981).

9. Bureau of Justice Statistics (1997).

10. Cook (1979). But see the critique in Kleck (1997).

11. See Zimring and Hawkins (1997) and Van Dijk and Mayhew (1993).

12. Zimring and Hawkins (1997).

13. Jana (1998, p. 8).

14. Cook (1987).

15. See Kleck and McElrath (1991), Zimring (1968), and Zimring (1972).

16. Saltzman et al. (1992).

17. See Wolfgang (1958) and Wright, Rossi, and Daly (1983).

18. See Zimring (1968), Zimring (1972), and Zimring and Hawkins (1997).

19. Cook (1987).

20. Ibid.

21. Anonymous message printed on a button.

22. Cook, Ludwig, and Hemenway (1997).

23. Cook (1991).

24. Kleck and Gertz (1995).

25. Sudman and Bradburn (1974).

26. Misreporting may occur because respondents report on events that occur outside the survey recall period (for example, reporting on events that occurred 13 months ago in response to questions about events during the last year) or because respondents unintentionally forget or misunderstand the question. Other forms of misreporting may be intentional, for example, because of the well-known tendency of respondents to present themselves in a favorable light to survey interviewers. Some respondents may view defensive gun use as a potentially illegal (and thus socially undesirable) behavior and, thus, not report their gun use. But at least some people view defensive gun use as a socially desirable behavior, as evidenced by the public reaction to the case of Dorothy Newton, who shot two robbers on the street in Richmond after having been wounded herself in a robbery one year earlier. A neighbor of Newton's remarked "Thank God someone finally stood up to the hoodlums around here. They think they run the city. Now I'm not saying that violence is a good answer to things. But too bad she didn't kill them both." The *Richmond Times Dispatch* wrote in an editorial: "The thought of cocky young predators scurrying like scalded dogs is one decent people find immensely satisfying." See Bowles (1996, p. A1) and Richmond Times-Dispatch (1996, p. A1).

27. Hemenway (1997a,b).

28. Reported in Hemenway (1997b).

29. See Cook, Ludwig, and Hemenway (1997) and Cook and Ludwig (1998).

30. Smith (1997).

31. Wright and Rossi (1994).

32. See, for example, Washington Post (1999a) and Washington Post (1999b).

33. Dykstra (1968) p. 121–148; cited in Wills (1999), p. 248–251.

34. Pierce and Bowers (1981).

35. Wright and Rossi (1994).

36. Rennison (1999).

37. Hill (1997).

38. Robuck-Mangum (1997).

39. See Black and Nagin (1998) and Ludwig (1998).

40. Lott and Mustard (1997).

41. See Black and Nagin (1998). Lott and Mustard attempt to address these omitted variables problems in a number of additional ways, although none of them appear to be successful. They include the area's burglary or robbery rate as a control variable in an attempt to control for unobserved local criminogenic effects, though in private correspondence Dan Black reports that these models also fail the specification test used in the Black and Nagin study. Lott and Mustard also estimate two-stage least squares (2SLS) models to control for omitted variables problems. Evidence that these 2SLS estimates are biased comes from their implausible magnitudes: the estimates suggest that shall-issue laws reduce homicides by 67%, rapes by 65%, and assaults by 73%. The implausible magnitudes of the 2SLS estimates is not immediately apparent from reading the Lott and Mustard paper because for some reason the authors report the implied effect of a one standard deviation increase in the probability of enacting a permissive concealed-carry law, rather than the implied effect of enacting such a law.

42. Ludwig (1998).

43. Cook and Leitzel (1996).

44. Kellermann et al. (1992).

45. Wintemute et al. (1999).

Chapter 4

1. Since 1989 the U.S. Office of Management and the Budget has required regulatory analysts to use willingness-to-pay-based estimates if they place a dollar value on saving lives (USOMB, 1989).

2. Since the program could make some people worse off, individual's WTP could be negative as well as positive.

3. Miller, Lestina, and Spicer (1998).

4. Harwood, Fountain, and Livermore (1998).

5. *The Seattle Times* (August 3, 1997) cites the CDC that the direct and indirect costs of asthma will reach approximately $14 billion in the next three years.

6. Collins (1999).

7. Weisbrod (1971) provides an early effort to estimate the social costs of polio, but he ignores the costs of prevention and avoidance.

8. Michael et al. (1994).

9. Rom (1997).

10. For further development of this idea, see Zeckhauser and Fisher (1995) and Berger et al. (1994).

11. Kahneman and Tversky (1979).

12. This approach to assessing the costs of illness and other social burdens has a long history. The first formal COI study was published as early as 1950. By 1980 over 200 such studies had been performed (Hu and Sandifer, 1981). Yet it has had critics from the beginning.

13. Hu and Sandifer, 1981. In 1967, Dorothy Rice codified this approach, and later, as head of the National Center for Health Statistics, she chaired a task force that issued *Guidelines for Cost of Illness Studies in the Public Health Services* (Hodgson and Meiners, 1979).

14. Rice, MacKenzie, and Associates (1989). Max and Rice (1993) applied this method to estimating the costs of gunshot violence.

15. Hodgson and Meiners (1982), p. 438.

16. Landefeld and Seskin (1982), p. 556.

17. Institute of Medicine (1981).

18. Schelling (1968); Mishan (1971).

19. Galanter and Luban (1993).

20. Schelling (1968), p. 127.

21. One limit on the amount that people are willing to expend to prolong their lives is the wish to leave a bequest. That may be particularly relevant in motivating suicides of elderly people facing the prospect of accumulating large bills for medical and nursing care.

22. See the discussion in Conley (1976) and Cook (1978).

23. See for example Smith and Gilbert (1984), Moore and Viscusi (1988a, 1988b, 1990a, 1990b), and Viscusi and Moore (1989).

24. See for example Portney (1981) and Gayer, Hamilton, and Viscusi (forthcoming).

25. For a comprehensive review see Viscusi (1993).

26. Viscusi (1993).

27. A great advantage of using market-price data, rather than data from surveys and other hypothetical exercises, is that market data are based on real choices made by people who have to reckon with a real possibility of injury or death.

28. Rosen (1986).

29. Two studies consider the risk premium in drug dealing: Levitt and Venkatesh (1998) and Reuter, MacCoun, and Murphy (1990).

30. Miller and Cohen (1997).

31. Thinking about how people whose behavior places them at high risk for suicide or homicide value their lives is complicated by the possibility that these values change over time. Terminal cancer patients apparently experience substantial fluctuations in their will to live (Chochinov et al., 1999), and people who lead dangerous lives as adolescents may later become working parents who feel a greater stake in preserving their well-being.

32. Viscusi (1998), p. 60.

33. Yet another problem with using generic estimates of the value of life is simply that the public does not see different causes of death as equivalent. Avoiding a microrisk of dying in a fire may be worth more for many than avoiding a microrisk of death by falling. The complications associated with extrapolating from one type of risk to another is known as the "benefits-transfer" problem; see, for example, Gayer, Hamilton, and Viscusi (forthcoming), and Viscusi, Hamilton, and Gayer (forthcoming).

34. These figures are taken from Miller and Cohen (1997), Table 4. For nonfatal gunshot wounds that result in a hospitalization, the jury award amount equals the subtotal for pain and suffering ($175,000) plus the productivity loss to physical and psychological injury ($42,799 + $81, or $42,880 in total), reported in 12/93 dollars (Ted Miller, personal communication).

35. Miller and Cohen use data from Jury Verdict Research (JVR), an organization that attempts to gather information on every civil suit that results in a jury award for personal injury. In the study from which Miller and Cohen (1996; 1997) draw their jury-award estimates, they report that the JVR database contains 1,467 jury awards for intentional injury during the period from 1980–1991, excluding wrongful death cases. By comparison, data from the National Crime Victimization Survey suggests that there are approximately 2.5 million violent crimes that result in injury each year, including attempted and completed rapes and sexual assaults (Rennison, 1999). Thus, there were around 27.5 million violent crimes that result in an injury during the 1980–1991 period, of which the JVR jury database represents around one-two-hundredth of one percent (1,467/27,500,000). These cases are likely to be more serious than average, even after controlling for different measurable aspects of the crime.

36. Cohen (1988), p. 540–541, quoting Bender (1986).

37. Cohen (1988), p. 541.

38. Another potential approach for valuing nonfatal injuries, suggested by economists David Cutler and Elizabeth Richardson Vigdor (Cutler and Richardson, 1997), is to use survey data to examine how people rate their quality of life with some health problem compared with perfect health. If, for example, people rate a year living with ar-

thritis as providing three-quarters as much utility as a year spent in perfect health, Cutler and Richardson value the costs per year of arthritis as one-quarter $(1 - 3/4 = 1/4)$ times the value of a year spent in perfect health (which they set at $100,000). One practical problem with this approach for our application is that the best available dataset for deriving respondent reports about self-perceived health status, the National Health Interview Survey, contains only a few gunshot injuries. As a result, in order to implement this approach we would be forced to assume that gunshot injuries have the same level of disutility as conditions that can be reliably studied using this dataset. But what conditions are "like" gunshot injuries? A related approach, is to ask physicians to rate the health consequences of life with some disease as compared to a year spent in perfect health (see Miller and Cohen, 1997), although to the best of our knowledge no such ratings are currently available for the quality of life for gunshot survivors.

39. For survey evidence on the importance of concern about others in risk valuation, see Viscusi, Magat, and Forrest (1988).

40. Diamond and Hausman (1994), p. 55, are dubious of this principle. Writing in the environmental policy context, they ask "if the government should devote more taxes to cleaning up lakes where neighbors are friendly with each other than to lakes where neighbors do not know (or care about) each other." While it may seem a bit strange, we believe that the answer is yes, and that as a practical matter (should no tax money be available for the purpose) the "friendly" lake community would have an easier time raising the funds for a cleanup than would the community of strangers.

41. Note that what is relevant here are *real*, not financial, resources. Money is just a means of keeping score. For example, someone with inherited wealth may be a net drain on the economy even though she lives within her (substantial) means, simply because she is consuming more than she is producing.

42. Swetnam (1980).

43. As far as we know, this calculation has never been attempted, so our assertion is decidedly speculative.

Chapter 5

1. Cook et al. (1999).

2. Lipscomb, Weinstein, and Torrance (1996). Economists convert streams of payments or costs incurred over time into a "present value" to reflect the fact that payments off into the future have less impact on current budgets than payments incurred today. For example, suppose that one's 18-year-old daughter starts college at Duke University tomorrow; the net change in the family budget for her freshman year equals $33,830, the listed price for tuition and room and board. Suppose

instead that we wish to calculate the present-value cost of freshman year at Duke for one's newborn infant. Assume for the moment that there is no inflation, and the costs of attending Duke for one year will remain $33,830 off into the foreseeable future. In this case, the family could pay for one year's worth of Duke tuition by investing only $19,900 today in a savings account that bears 3% interest per year—when the child turns 18, the $19,900 will have grown to equal the necessary amount. Thus, a $33,830 cost 18 years off into the future has a present value below this amount because a lesser sum could be invested and accrue interest over time.

3. Estimates for annual medical expenses (including nursing home costs) for men and women are calculated from the National Health Interview Survey by University of Chicago economist Willard Manning and his colleagues. See Manning et al. (1991).

4. People at high risk for gunshot injury presumably have lower-than-average rates of health insurance coverage because of their below-average socioeconomic status (documented in Chapter 2), combined with the association between socioeconomic status and health access in the United States. Rowland, Feder, and Keenan (1998); Fronstin (1998); Lillie-Blanton et al. (1999).

5. We may be concerned that one specific group at high risk of gunshot injury—those with chronic or terminal ailments, which in turn appears to contribute to an elevated risk of suicide (Chapter 2)—may have above-average lifetime medical expenses. Yet calculations by Christina Clark, a graduate student in public policy at Georgetown University, suggest that the counterfactual medical costs for those with poor health at the time of their self-inflicted injuries turn out to be quite close to those for all gun-suicide victims. Data from the 1993 National Mortality Followback Survey (Appendix A) are used to estimate the different health ailments that afflict the 30 to 40% of gun-suicide victims who are in poor health at the time of their injuries, which are then matched with the estimated lifetime costs of these conditions. For example, an estimated 11% of gun suicide victims in 1993 had some form of cancer at the time of their gunshot injury. While we have very limited information about the nature of each patient's cancer, data from the American Cancer Society suggest that the average treatment cost per cancer patient equals $31,500 (in 1998 dollars). Similarly, around 3% of gun suicide victims have Alzheimer's or some other form of dementia or organic brain disorder, with the average lifetime cost of treating Alzheimer's disease estimated at $174,000 (1998 dollars). Around 4% of gun suicide victims have had a stroke in the past. Since approximately one-third of all stroke survivors have another stroke within three years, we estimate that 1.3% of gun suicide victims would have had another stroke, with an average treatment cost equal to $51,200 in 1998 dollars (National

Stroke Association). Finally, around 11% of gun suicide victims have a lung condition such as emphysema or bronchitis. While data on the treatment costs for these diseases is quite limited, under some reasonable assumptions, we calculate the average costs per patient to equal $2,210. According to the National Heart, Lung, and Blood Institute of the National Institutes of Health (1999), there are 1.9 million Americans with emphysema at any point in time. Total annual expenditures for the treatment of emphysema are $2.5 billion, or around $1,300 per patient. NIH figures also suggest that 59% of those admitted to the intensive care unit with emphysema die within one year. We assume that the average life expectancy of acute emphysema patients who would attempt gun suicide is $(1.0 / 0.59) = 1.7$ years. As a result, the average costs per emphysema patient is assumed to be $2,210, which we also assume holds for those with bronchitis. Unfortunately, the NMFS data do not enable us to determine whether decedents who had bronchitis before their death had serious or less-serious cases of this disease. An additional 10 or 11% of gun suicide victims in the NMFS show signs of poor health (bedridden, unable to leave the house), but we cannot identify the specific health problem from which they suffer. We assume that the distribution of illnesses for this group is the same as the distribution of illnesses for the 30% of chronically ill gun suicide victims for whom we can identify their illness. The average estimated lifetime costs for this group in poor health is thus around $35,000, quite close to the figure reported in the text for all gun-suicide victims.

6. The same analysis should hold when an employed worker suffers a permanent total disability due to gunshot wound; since such cases may constitute only a relatively small share of all gunshot wounds, we ignore them in our analysis.

7. Even people who are employed in the "black" or "gray" markets may also be replaced by immigration or from people within the local economy. Another complication that arises in thinking about worker-replacement issues arises because some gunshot victims may be unemployed at the time of their injuries, but would have entered the labor force in the future. In these cases, the victim is replaced in the job he would have taken in the future by either an immigrant or an unemployed local. Since almost nothing is known about the lifetime employment trajectories of those who experience a period of high risk for gunshot injury, we make the simplifying assumption that victims who are employed at their death would have been employed throughout their lives, and those who are not employed would never have worked had they not been shot. Since this assumption probably understates the amount of worker replacement (and thus overstates the medical savings that we net out), our assumption is conservative and leads us to understate net medical costs.

Chapter 6

1. Rice & MacKenzie (1989), p. 70.

2. For example, Rice and MacKenzie (1989); Max and Rice (1993); Miller and Cohen (1996); Miller and Cohen (1997).

3. The best available evidence suggests that differences in standardized achievement test scores explains most (but not all) of the differences in earnings across groups; for example, economists Derek Neal and William Johnson find that controlling for high school test scores explains three-quarters of the wage difference between African-American and white men, and all of the wage difference between African-American and white women (Neal and Johnson, 1996).

4. We obtain qualitatively similar findings for women, which are not presented in order to simplify the exposition.

5. We include estimates for lost household production for men and women to make our estimates comparable to those obtained in previous cost-of-illness studies. Our estimates for the value of household production come from figures calculated by Expectancy Data of Shawnee Mission, Kansas. See Expectancy Data (1999).

6. Rice & MacKenzie (1989); Max and Rice (1993), and Miller and Cohen (1996, 1997).

7. Our procedure still probably overstates the lost earnings due to gun violence, because gunshot victims probably have below-average life expectancies compared with other people of the same sex, age, race, and schooling. For example, many gun homicide victims seem to lead quite risky lives (as evidenced by their previous criminal records), while many gun suicide victims appear to suffer from chronic or terminal illnesses prior to suffering their gunshot injuries.

8. The central insight that net rather than gross consumption is of primary interest was emphasized by Northwestern economist Burton Weisbrod as far back as the early 1960s. Weisbrod (1961).

9. Engen and Gale (1997).

10. Hodgkinson et al (1996).

11. Criminological research suggests that the average criminal career ranges from between 5 and 15 years, while the number of crimes committed per individual is sharply skewed—most offenders commit only a few crimes a year, though the most criminally active 10% may commit 100 or more. See Blumstein et al. (1986).

Chapter 7

1. Thanks to Arthur Kellermann and Daniel Webster for pushing us to focus on the effects of gun violence on the criminal justice system.

2. See Zimring (1968) and Cook (1991).

3. For example, data from a sample survey of state felony convictions

(the National Judicial Reporting Program) and a census of federal convictions (the Federal Justice Statistics Program) show that in 1996, the most recent year for which such data are available, there were over 11,000 people sentenced to prison or jail for murder and over 50,000 people incarcerated for aggravated assault (Brown 1999). Thus for every homicide reported to the police, 0.57 people will be incarcerated, with an expected prison or jail time equal to nearly 11 years on average. In contrast, had these attacks instead result in nonfatal injuries to the victim, all of which we assume would ultimately become known to the police, only 1 perpetrator in 20 would ultimately be incarcerated, with an expected sentence of just over 3 years. (Our estimates for the number of homicides known to the police come from the FBI's Uniform Crime Reporting [UCR] system, reported in 1996 [FBI, 1997].) Sentence length information is the product of the mean sentence length imposed on those convicted of homicide and sentenced to jail and the percent of sentence that these prisoners are expected to ultimately serve (see Brown, 1999).

4. Juveniles who commit homicides are also far more likely to be waived in to the adult justice system and thus receive longer prison sentences than those who are arrested for aggravated assault (Dawson, 1992; Zimring, 1998). This difference will be captured by our ratio of felony convictions to crimes reported in Table 7.1, though our calculations ignore the additional costs arising from the more severe punishments that the juvenile justice system metes out to teens under its jurisdiction who are adjudicated delinquent for homicide rather than aggravated assault. Another complication stems from the possibility that the number of perpetrators per crime may be somewhat different for homicides and aggravated assaults, but such a difference should be reflected in differences across crimes in the number of incarcerations per crime.

5. See Cook and Leitzel (1996).

6. See also the last two columns of Table C2 in Appendix C.

7. In fact, concern about losses in class time motivated the Los Angeles public school system to decide against screening each student on the way into school, despite the city's high rates of gun violence. See Firestone (1999).

8. The Chicago public school system Bureau of Safety and Security reports that 994 personnel are employed as watchmen, security officers, and security aids, with average annual salaries of $11,000, $17,000 and $20,000, respectively. While the distribution of employees across jobs is not available, we assume an average salary of around $17,000; with a 44% fringe-benefit rate in the city, the total average expense comes to around $25,000.

9. The Bureau of Safety and Security reports that these Security Supervisors work no more than 20 hours per week at an hourly wage of $15 per hour, so the monthly salary cost is $1,200 plus 44% fringe benefit rate bringing the total to around $1,700 per month. We assume

these officers work a 9-month academic year, bringing the annual cost to $15,500.

10. The Chicago Police Department reports that police officers earn between $33,500 and $59,200 per year, for an average of around $46,000, which we then multiply by 1.44 to account for fringe benefits.

11. This range comes from a survey conducted by Heath Einstein of nine manufacturers of such vests, using retail prices listed on the world wide web.

12. This estimate comes from multiplying the total number of police protection employees (856,000) times one-fifth (on average the proportion whose vests are replaced in any given year) times $550, the midpoint of the price range for bulletproof Kevlar vests. This figure assumes that every police-protection employee is already assigned their own vest and that each police department rotates vests once every five years. While the actual annual expenditure level may be slightly different, our estimate of $100 million is probably in the right ballpark.

13. Laband and Sophocleus (1992) report a 1985 cost per passenger screen equal to $0.79, which, when converted to 1998 dollars using the Consumer Price Index, is around $1.20.

14. U.S. Bureau of the Census (1999a), Table 1070.

15. Ibid, Table 1075.

16. Noble (1999).

17. Cullen and Levitt (1999).

18. Urban economists believe that these "agglomeration economies" may stem from a number of possible sources: Firms in the same industry that locate near each other may experience lower costs of acquiring (transporting) intermediate inputs; face-to-face interactions between people in different firms may be easier in the central city, which in turn facilitates the transfer of knowledge and promotes economic growth (see Glaeser, 1995, and Ihlanfeldt, 1995). Some suggestive empirical evidence to support this hypothesis comes from evidence that information-processing firms tend to locate in the city and that suburban and city growth rates are positively correlated (Ihlanfeldt, 1995). The vitality of the central city may affect the overall region's economic health in other ways as well, as discussed in Ihlanfeldt (1995). For example, national perceptions of the metropolitan area may be heavily influenced by the conditions of the urban center, which in turn affects the decisions by firms and people to relocate there. Cities may contain amenities (such as museums or baseball stadiums) that are used by people throughout the area, so a deterioration in the condition of the city makes these less attractive and thereby lowers the quality of life in the area. City and suburban residents, and even people who live outside of the metropolitan area, may derive value from the sense of community that a thriving central city provide. Finally, there is the possibility that the financial problems of cities may spread to suburbs.

19. Wilson (1987).

20. See Ludwig, Duncan, and Hirschfield (2001) and Ludwig, Duncan, and Pinkston (1999).

21. Hamermesh (1998) estimates that a 75% reduction in homicide would increase welfare by $4 to $10 billion per year. The figure per homicide comes from dividing these annual gains by 75% of the annual number of homicides in the United States, equal to 18,209 in 1997 (Federal Bureau of Investigation, 1998).

22. These figures are calculated as follows: since around one-fifth of all assault-related gunshot injuries are fatal (Chapter 2) and the case-fatality rate of nongun assaults is around one-third as high (Cook and Leitzel, 1996), then every 100 gunshot injuries that are averted prevents 13 homicides. Our figure per gunshot injury comes from calculating the increased productivity associated with the elimination of 100 gunshot injuries (equal to 13 times the productivity loss per homicide), and then dividing by 100.

23. Halbfinger (1998, p. A1).

24. Manning et al. (1991).

25. Thanks to Jeffrey Conte for these anecdotes.

26. Thomas (1993).

Chapter 8

1. Schelling (1968, p. 143).

2. Ibid.

3. Hausman, Leonard, and McFadden (1993).

4. Desvousges et al. (1993).

5. Shavell (1993).

6. Arrow et al. (1993).

7. Mitchell and Carson (1989).

8. See also Paul Portney (1994) for a summary of the NOAA panel recommendations.

9. See Hamermesh (1998) and Cullen and Levitt (1999).

10. Sudman and Bradburn (1974).

11. See, for example, Kahneman and Knetsch (1992). The "purchase of moral satisfaction" is sometimes also known as the purchase of "warm glow" (from the feeling that people purportedly receive from supporting a worthwhile cause). Some proponents of cv decidedly reject this possibility: " 'Warm glow' is simply a red herring. I have seen no empirical evidence that people get a warm glow from voting to raise their own taxes, whether in real life or in a contingent valuation study" (Hanemann, 1994, p. 33).

12. Hanemann (1994).

13. See Kahneman and Knetcsch (1992) and Desvousges et al. (1993).

14. Hanemann (1994).

15. For conflicting views, see Diamond and Hausman (1993 and 1994), in contrast to Hanemann (1994).

16. Hanemann (1994).

17. See Hausman (1993), Hanemann (1994), and Diamond and Hausman (1994).

18. Hanemann (1994).

19. See, for example, Cutler and Richardson (1998) and Miller and Cohen (1996, 1997).

20. For more details about the survey, see Kuby, Imhof, and Shin (1999).

21. Hamermesh (1998).

22. The results for overall violent crimes are reported in Cullen and Levitt (1999). Unpublished estimates specific to homicide were kindly provided to us by Julie Cullen and Steve Levitt.

23. Schelling (1968) argues that "Furthermore, this [decision about individual health risks] is, more than most decisions, a family one, not an individual one. . . . The family gets little attention in economics. It is an income-sharing unit, a consumption-sharing unit, and a welfare-sharing unit. That is, they live off the same income, share the same bathroom, and care about each other" (p. 145).

24. One implication of this assumption is that our analysis should convert the NGPS sampling weights from person weights into household weights. The NGPS respondent weights calculated by NORC equal one divided by the probability of the household's selection into the sample. The weights are then divided by the adult's probability of selection from within the household, equal to (1/A) where A is the number of adults in the home. To convert these into household weights we multiply by (1/A).

25. U.S. Bureau of the Census (1997).

26. Since only 2.2% of all marriages were interracial in 1992, the last year for which such data are available (U.S. Bureau of the Census, 1999a), we infer "household race" from the respondent's race.

27. This can be seen most easily by way of a simple model in which there are two communities, A and B, populated by people with identical incomes and preferences. Assume that everyone in this society works in area B, that the costs of commuting from area A to B equals $10, that residents in both communities are all renters, and that landlords live someplace else. If housing markets are competitive, the rental rates in areas A and B should adjust such that people are indifferent between living in either of the two communities in equilibrium; we assume that in the absence of gun violence, the rental rates would equal $90 and $100, respectively. Now suppose that the risk of gun violence is 1/100,000 in area A, and 2/100,000 in area B, and that people in this society are willing to pay $5 to avoid a 1/100,000 risk of gunshot injury. If the risks of gunshot injury are fully capitalized in rents, in equilibrium the

new rent in areas A and B will equal $90 and $95, respectively, and no one in either community will relocate in response to the introduction of gun violence. It is easy to see that the residents of area A will be willing to pay $5 to eliminate the threat of gun violence in this society. Perhaps less intuitive is the observation that residents of area B will pay only $5 as well, even though they face a 2/100,000 risk of gunshot injury. The reason is that the elimination of gun violence produces a benefit to B residents of $10, which is partially offset by a $5 increase in rent that they would experience.

28. See Viscusi (1993), whose range we have converted into 1998 dollars.

29. This comes from multiplying twice the highest estimate for workplace injuries reported in Viscusi (1993), around $300,000 in 1998 dollars, by the number of nonfatal gun injuries for every fatality (4), and subtracting this figure ($1.2 million) from the estimated value of 5 gun injuries ($5 million).

30. Anderson (1999).

31. Zimring and Hawkins (1997).

32. For example, Hamermesh (1998) finds that a city's homicide rate affects the amount of evening and night work that occurs in the metropolitan area, but nonfatal crimes have little effect on work behavior. Similarly, Cullen and Levitt (1999) find that homicides have a much larger effect on population flight from cities than do other crimes. (Unpublished calculations for the effects of homicide on city population loss were kindly provided to us by Julie Berry Cullen and Steve Levitt.)

33. The range for the workplace-study estimates arises from different assumptions about weapon substitution and differences in risk preferences between gunshot victims and others in the population; see Appendix D for details.

34. Levitt and Venkatesh (1998).

35. Miller and Hemenway (1999).

36. Thanks to Will Manning for this point.

Chapter 9

1. Cook, Molliconi, and Cole (1995); Cook and Ludwig (1996).

2. Cook, Molliconi, and Cole (1995), Sheley and Wright (1993), Wright and Rossi (1994), Ash et al. (1996).

3. Cook, Molliconi, and Cole (1995).

4. Weil and Knox (1996).

5. Cook, Molliconi, and Cole (1995), p. 65.

6. Wright and Rossi (1994).

7. Wright, Wintemute, and Rivara (1999).

8. The follow-up arrest rates for both groups in the study by Wright

and her colleagues were fairly low, and only 3% of these violent-crime arrests were for homicide. If we project the results of this study to the 44,000 applicants who were denied their application to purchase a handgun in 1996 in the 32 states that were subject to the new background-check requirements imposed by the 1994 Federal Brady Act, the result is a prediction of just eight fewer homicides and perhaps another 30 or so nonfatal gunshot wounds.

9. Ludwig and Cook (2000).

10. A study by Doug Weil (1997) provides some evidence to suggest that the Federal Brady Act reduced illicit gun trafficking from states with lax regulations to those with more stringent regulations.

11. Kleck (1984).

12. Loftin et al. (1991).

13. Britt, Bordua, and Kleck (1986) have criticized the use of the suburbs as a control group since the socioeconomic characteristics of the two areas are quite different, and they note that the reduction in gun homicides in Washington closely mirrored the drop found in a comparable local city that did not ban handguns—Baltimore. The similarity in the trends for gun homicide between Washington and Baltimore seem to point to causes other than D.C.'s handgun ban as an explanation for the drop in both cities. Yet there are also important differences between the patterns in D.C. and Baltimore that lead us to conclude that the Washington reduction is plausibly the result at least in part of the handgun ban. For example, McDowall, Loftin, and Wiersema (1995) note that in Washington, there was a decrease in gun homicides but not for nongun homicides following the handgun ban. In contrast, in Baltimore both gun and nongun homicides decreased, which suggests that a different process (perhaps a general reduction in criminogenic factors) is responsible for the drop in gun homicides. Gun *suicides* also declined in Washington, which did not occur in Baltimore. The frequency of gun suicides should plausibly be affected by a gun ban but be less sensitive to criminogenic factors that may affect homicide trends in both cities. Finally, McDowall and colleagues note that neither gun homicides nor gun suicides decreased during this period in Boston or Memphis, the two cities with 1990 populations just above and below that of Washington, D.C. (McDowall, Loftin, and Wiersema, 1995).

14. Gun homicide rates eventually increased dramatically in Washington, D.C. starting in the mid-1980s, as the crack epidemic that hit other large cities also affected the District. That gun homicide rates increased sharply during this period in Washington is not in itself evidence that the handgun ban was ineffective, since the relevant comparison is to what the increase *would have been* in the city had the gun ban *not* been in effect.

15. Dvorak (1999).

16. Posted on the MSNBC electronic bulletin board, August 24, 1999.

17. Sherman, Shaw, and Rogan (1995).

18. Indianapolis implemented a similar program in the East and North districts of the city beginning in 1995. In the East district, police stopped vehicles for traffic violations, issued warning citations, and where probable cause existed, searched the vehicle for illegal guns. In the North district, police followed the original Kansas City Gun Experiment design and focused on stopping cars that were "suspicious" based on a developed profile. Violent crimes decreased in the North district but increased slightly in the East district (OJJDP, 1999). Determining whether these changes are due to the police patrols is complicated by the fact that other parts of the city cannot be used as control areas, since other antiviolence programs (such as community policing) were implemented in other districts.

19. Sherman, Shaw, and Rogan (1995) report that the program required 4,512 person-hours of targeted police resources to implement. Since the average costs of each additional patrol officer is on the order of $80,000 for salary plus overhead and support expenses (Levitt, 1997), if we assume that a full-time police officer works 2,000 hours per year then the costs of these additional patrols is around $180,000.

20. Cook and Ludwig (1996).

21. That is, Cummings et al. (1997) include year dummies to control for variation over time in national rates for unintentional shootings and state fixed-effects to control for constant differences across states in the rate of unintentional gunshot injuries to children.

22. Webster and Starnes (1999).

23. From Appendix D, we estimate that the costs of unintentional gunshot wounds are somewhere between $130,000 and $320,000 per injury. In 1997, there were 142 fatal unintentional shootings to children under the age of 15 in the United States so a 41% reduction equals 58 fatalities. The statistics presented in Chapter 2 suggest that around 7% of all unintentional shootings are fatal, a case-fatality rate that would imply that safe storage laws prevent nearly 830 unintentional shootings altogether (fatal plus nonfatal).

24. The 1994 National Survey of Private Ownership of Firearms (NSPOF), discussed in Cook and Ludwig (1996), asks a nationally representative sample of adults whether they have a gun in the home, and whether they have children under 18 in the home. The NSPOF also asks respondents whether any guns in the home are stored "unlocked and loaded." The responses to the NSPOF imply that 5 million households have both children and at least one gun stored both unlocked *and* loaded. Unfortunately, the NSPOF does not enable us to identify the number of households with children that have at least one gun stored

either unlocked or unloaded. (While respondents with guns in the home are asked a follow-up question about the storage practices of one randomly selected gun from the household's gun stock, the answers to this question also do not enable us to precisely answer the question of interest.)

25. See, for example, Schiller (1998).

26. Kessler and Levitt (1999). The average sentence enhancement imposed from Proposition 8 is difficult to determine—the law required that "all 'serious' felony offenders . . . receive a 5-year enhancement for each prior conviction of a 'serious' felony offense or a 1-year enhancement for each prior prison term served for any offense, whichever was greater. In addition, Proposition 8 expanded the scope and severity of the enhancements by eliminating the statute of limitations . . . that only considered a defendant's record for at most the past 10 years, by prohibiting judges from sentencing defendants to serve their enhancements concurrently with their base sentence and by requiring that each of the enhancements be served consecutively" (p. 353).

27. McDowall, Loftin, and Wiersema (1992). The authors find an effect of these sentencing enhancement laws equal to 0.69 of a standard deviation in each city's monthly homicide count; using the monthly mean and standard deviations for Detroit, one of the cities in their sample, this translates to a 14% reduction in homicides. This is comparable in magnitude to the effect of 20% found by Kessler and Levitt (1999), even though Proposition 8 in California only applied to repeat offenders and imposed additional penalties that varied with the arrestees previous criminal history.

28. Donohue and Siegelman (1998).

29. Downloaded from National Rifle Association, Institute for Legislation Action web page (NRA, 2000).

30. Torry (1999); Janofsky (1999); NRA (2000); and material downloaded from Virginians Against Handgun Violence (VAHV, 2000).

31. Our calculation is derived as follows: FBI data indicate that there were 112 homicides in Richmond in 1996 (FBI, 1997). Other reports indicate that the proportion of all homicides that involved firearms in Richmond in 1997 equaled 87% (Schiller, 1998), implying that there were around 97 gun homicides in Richmond in 1996. Since the case-fatality rate for assault-related gunshot injuries is between 15 and 20% (see Cook, 1985), the gun-homicide figure implies that there must have been somewhere between 500 and 600 gunshot injuries altogether in Richmond in 1996. Since Project Exile was in effect for around two years as of March 14, 1999, if there were 500 gunshot injuries in 1996 and the program reduces gun violence by 15% then the benefits are on the order of $150 million (75 fewer gun injuries per year, times our estimated benefits of around $1 million per gunshot injury averted). If instead the program reduces gun violence by 20% and there are 600 gunshot in-

juries in Richmond in 1996, the program has benefits on the order of $240 million.

32. Note that to the extent that the program has a deterrent effect, the net incarceration cost is reduced because the flow of new defendants is reduced. If the deterrent effect is large enough, then the net cost may be zero or even negative.

33. Downloaded from National Rifle Association web page (NRA, 1999).

34. In the short-run there may be an increase in production of such technologies prior to the ban that floods the market, thus minimizing the initial effects of the policy.

35. Cook (1981b).

36. NRA (1999).

37. Roth and Koper (1997).

38. Nader (1965).

39. GAO (1991); see also Vernick et al. (1999).

40. Magazine safeties prevent semi-automatic pistols or rifles from being fired when the magazine that holds the ammunition is removed from the gun, thereby preventing the operator from mistakenly discharging the weapon with the magazine removed in the belief that the gun is unloaded; see Vernick et al. (1999).

41. Cook, Molliconi, and Cole (1995); Cook and Ludwig (1996).

42. Teret, Webster, Vernick et al. (1998).

43. Bai (1999).

44. Johns Hopkins Center for Gun Policy and Research (1999).

45. O'Connell (1999) and Reuters (2000b).

46. Johns Hopkins Center for Gun Policy and Research (1999).

47. Cook (1981a).

48. Teret, Webster, Vernick et al. (1998).

49. Jacobs and Potter (1999).

50. Cook, Molliconi, and Cole (1995); but see also Jacobs and Potter (1995).

51. Under this system, when a gun turns up at a crime scene, police would still be able to trace the ownership path of the gun, starting with the original owner's own record (who under the current regulatory system is already on record with an FFL). The owner in this case would be required to produce evidence that the gun had been legally transferred through an FFL to someone who passed a background check (in which case police repeat the process with the next owner) or, if evidence of such a transfer is not produced, the most recent owner of record is held liable in some way.

52. Bonnie et al. (1999).

53. Interestingly, our proposals are quite similar to those offered by Gary Kleck (1997) in his book *Targeting Guns*, even though his research is often used by opponents of gun control measures.

Appendix A

1. See NCHS (1999); Annest et al. (1996); NCHS (1988).
2. U.S. Bureau of the Census (1986).
3. See Annest, Mercy, Gibson, and Ryan (1995) and Davis, Annest, Powell, and Mercy (1996).
4. Davis, Annest, Powell, and Mercy (1996).
5. May et al. (1999).

Appendix B

1. Our estimates for the costs of treating gunshot victims are the result of a collaborative project with Ted Miller and Bruce Lawrence; several of these findings were published previously as: "The Medical Costs of Gunshot Injuries in the United States." Philip J. Cook, Bruce Lawrence, Jens Ludwig, and Ted R. Miller, *Journal of the American Medical Association* 282, no. 5 (August 4, 1999): 447–454.
2. Finkler (1982).
3. Annest et al. (1995).
4. Brick, Tourangeau, and Cantor (1992); Davis et al. (1996).
5. Miller et al. (1995).
6. Miller and Cohen (1996); Miller and Cohen (1997).
7. Miller et al. (1995).
8. Bureau of the Census (1996).
9. Miller, Luchter, and Brinkman (1989).
10. DeVivo (1997).
11. HCFA (1999).
12. Roberts et al. (1999).
13. Miller and Cohen (1996; 1997).
14. Miller and Cohen (1997).
15. National Highway Transportation Safety Administration (1983).
16. Cook (1979, 1985, 1987, 1991).
17. Cook (1991); Cook and Leitzel (1996).
18. See for example Miller and Cohen (1997).
19. We estimate the proportion of gun homicide victims in 1993 who worked during the year before death to be 0.66 using data from the 1993 National Mortality Followback Survey (NMFS, 1999).
20. Using data from the 1993 NMFS, we estimate the proportion of victims of fatal unintentional shootings who worked in the year before death to be 0.62.
21. We estimate the proportion of gun suicide victims in 1993 who were working during the year before death to be 0.52 using data from the 1993 NMFS.
22. See Fronstin (1998). The sources of payment for the victim's gunshot injuries may be different from the payers for the medical expenses

he would have incurred had he not been shot. Some nonelderly victims who are unemployed (and thus uninsured) at the time of their gunshot injuries would have eventually taken jobs, and their medical expenses would be covered by private health insurance. Of course, the opposite scenario is also possible: some people may be shot while they are working and covered by private health insurance, though the bulk of the medical expenses they would have incurred had they not been shot come when they are old and covered by Medicaid.

23. Fronstin (1998) actually reports that 18% of Americans were without health insurance (Table 1, page 4). In his table, CPS respondents can have more than one source of coverage, so we assume that the 4% of people who report either private health insurance and government and "no health insurance" are actually covered by either private or government programs.

Appendix C

1. Rice, MacKenzie, and Associates (1989), Max and Rice (1993), and Miller and Cohen (1996, 1997).

2. Keil et al. (1992); Feinstein (1993); Sorlie, Backlund, and Keller (1995); LeClere, Rogers, and Peters (1997).

Appendix D

1. See Cameron and James (1987) and Cameron (1988).
2. Hanemann, Loomis, and Kanninen (1991).
3. Yates (1981).
4. Maddala (1977).
5. Manning (1998).
6. Cameron and Quiggin (1994).
7. Ibid.
8. Alberini (1995).
9. Mitchell and Carson (1989).
10. Freeman (1993).
11. Miller and Cohen (1996, 1997).
12. See, for example, Miller and Cohen (1996, 1997) for an application of this methodology to the case of gunshot injuries.
13. Tolley, Kenkel, and Fabian (1994).
14. Cutler and Richardson (1997).
15. Heinzerling (1998).
16. Revesz (1999).
17. Viscusi (1993).
18. Viscusi (1998).
19. Miller and Hemenway (1999).
20. Thanks to Will Manning for this point.

21. Viscusi and Evans (1990).

22. See Miller and Cohen (1996, 1997).

23. Miller and Cohen (1996).

24. As noted above, we adjust column (3) for differences in attitudes toward risk among the population at highest risk of gunshot injury by multiplying by 0.4, which is the ratio of the estimated value of a statistical life for workers in high-risk jobs, divided by the value obtained from more general samples of workers.

References

Alberini, Anna. 1995. Efficiency vs. Bias of Willingness-to-Pay Estimates: Bivariate and Interval-Data Models. *Journal of Environmental Economics and Management* 29: 169–80.

Anderson, David A. 1999. The Aggregate Burden of Crime. *Journal of Law and Economics* 42 (2): 611–42.

Annest, Joseph L., James A. Mercy, Delinda R. Gibson, and George W. Ryan. 1995. National Estimates of Nonfatal Firearm-Related Injuries: Beyond the Tip of the Iceberg. *Journal of the American Medical Association* 273 (22): 1749–54.

Arrow, Kenneth, et al. 1993. Report of the NOAA Panel on Contingent Valuation. *Federal Register* (Washington, D.C.), February 15, 41

Ash, Peter, Arthur L. Kellermann, Dawna Fuqua-Whitley, and Amri Johnson. 1996. Gun Acquisition and Use by Juvenile Offenders. *Journal of the American Medical Association* 275 (22): 1754–58.

Bai, Matt. 1999. Finally, Smart Guns for Sale. December 10. www.Newsweek.com.

Bender, Matthew. 1986. *Damages in Tort Actions*. New York: Matthew Bender.

Berger, Mark, Glenn Blomquist, Donald Kenkel, and George Tolley. 1994. Framework for Valuing Health Risks. In *Valuing Health for Policy: An Economic Approach*, ed. George Tolley, Donald Kenkel, and Robert Fabian, 23–41. Chicago: University of Chicago Press.

Black, Dan, and Daniel Nagin. 1998. Do 'Right to Carry' Laws Reduce Violent Crime? *Journal of Legal Studies* 27 (1): 209–19.

Blumstein, Alfred. 1995. Youth Gun Violence, Guns, and the Illicit-Drug Industry. *Journal of Criminal Law and Criminology* 86: 10–36.

Blumstein, Alfred, Jacqueline Cohen, Jeffrey A. Roth, and Christy A. Visher. 1986. *Criminal Careers and "Career Criminals."* Vol. 1. Washington, D.C.: National Academy Press.

Bonnie, Richard J., Carolyn E. Fulco, and Catharyn T. Liverman. 1999. Magnitude and Costs. In *Reducing the Burden of Injury: Advancing Prevention and Treatment*, ed. Richard J. Bonnie, Carolyn E. Fulco, and Catharyn T. Liverman, 42–43. Washington, D.C.: National Academy Press.

Bowles, Scott. 1996. A Gun at Her Head Forced Her Hand. *Washington Post*, June 28, A1.

Brick, M., K. Tourangeau, and D. Cantor. 1992. *A Statistical Evaluation and Cost Assessment of Using the National Electronic Injury Surveillance System (NEISS) to Obtain National Estimates of Nonfatal Firearm Injuries*. Rockville, Md.: Westat.

Britt, Chester L., David J. Bordua, and Gary Kleck. 1996. A Reassessment of the D.C. Gun Law: Some Cautionary Notes on the Use of Interrupted Time Series Designs for Policy Impact Assessment. *Law and Society Review* 30 (2): 361–79.

Brooke, James. 1999a. Diary of a High School Gunman Reveals a Plan to Kill Hundreds. *New York Times*, April 27, A1.

———. 1999b. Terror in Littleton: The Overview. *New York Times*, April 21, A1.

Brown, Jodi M. 1999. *Felony Sentences in the United States, 1996*. Washington, D.C.: U.S. Department of Justice, Bureau of Justice Statistics.

Bureau of Justice Statistics. 1997. *Crime Victimization in the United States, 1994: A National Crime Victimization Survey Report*. Washington, D.C.: U.S. Department of Justice.

Cameron, Trudy Ann. 1988. A New Paradigm for Valuing Non-Market Goods Using Referendum Data: Maximum Likelihood Estimation by Censored Logistic Regression. *Journal of Environmental Economics and Management* 15: 355–79.

Cameron, Trudy Ann, and Michelle D. James. 1987. Efficient Estimation Methods for 'Closed Ended' Contingent Valuation Surveys. *Review of Economics and Statistics* 69: 269–76.

Cameron, Trudy Ann, and John Quiggin. 1994. Estimation Using Contingent Valuation Data from a 'Dichotomous Choice with Follow-Up' Questionnaire. *Journal of Environmental Economics and Management* 27: 218–34.

Cannon, Angie et al. 1999. Why? *U.S. News and World Report*, May 3.

Centers for Disease Control. 1996a. *Inventory of Federal Data Systems in the United States for Injury Surveillance, Research and Prevention Activities*. J. L. Annest, J. M. Conn, and S. P. James investigators, Atlanta, Ga.: *National Center for Injury Prevention and Control*, Centers for Disease Control.

———. 1996b. Mortality Data. 1996 Mortality Rates from Unintentional Injuries. Available: *www.cdc.gov/ncipc Atlanta*. Accessed July 10, 1999.

Chochinov, Harvey Max, Douglas Tataryn, Jennifer J. Clinch, and Deborah Dudgeon. 1999. Will to Live in the Terminally Ill. *The Lancet* 354: 816–19.

Clotfelter, Charles T., and John C. Hahn. 1978. Assessing the 55 m.p.h. National Speed Limit. *Policy Sciences* 9 (June): 281–94.

Cohen, Mark A. 1988. Pain, Suffering, and Jury Awards: A Study of the Costs of Crime to Victims. *Law and Society Review* 22 (3): 537–55.

Collins, Huntly. 1999. Iron Lungs and Isolation: Tales of the Polio Years. Available: *www.philly.com/packages/polio/text//surv23.asp*. Accessed February 23, 1999.

Conley, Brian C. 1976. The Value of Human Life in the Demand for Safety. *American Economic Review* 66 (March): 45–55.

Cook, Philip J. 1978. The Value of Human Life in the Demand for Safety: Comment. *American Economic Review* 68 (4): 710–11.

———. 1979. The Effect of Gun Availability on Robbery and Robbery Murder: A Cross-Section Study of Fifty Cities. *Policy Studies Review Annual* 3: 743–81.

———. (1981a). Guns and Crime: The Power of Long Division. *Journal of Policy Analysis and Management* (Fall): 120–25.

———. 1981b. The 'Saturday Night Special': An Assessment of Alternative Definitions from a Policy Perspective. *Journal of Criminal Law and Criminology* 72, no. 4 (Winter): 1735–45.

———. 1985. The Case of the Missing Victims: Gunshot Woundings in the National Crime Survey. *Journal of Quantitative Criminology* 1 (1): 91–102.

———. 1987. Robbery Violence. *Journal of Criminal Law and Criminology* 70 (2).

———. 1991. The Technology of Personal Violence. In *Crime and Justice: An Annual Review of Research*, ed. M. Tonry, 1–71. Chicago: University of Chicago Press.

Cook, Philip J., and James Blose. 1981. State Programs for Screening Handgun Buyers. *Annals of the American Academy of Political and Social Science*, May: 80–91.

Cook, Philip J., and J. H. Laub. 1998. The Unprecedented Epidemic of Youth Violence. In *Crime and Justice: An Annual Review of Research*, ed. M. H. Moore and M. Tonry, 26–64. Chicago: University of Chicago Press.

Cook, Philip J., B. Lawrence, Jens Ludwig, and Ted R. Miller. 1999. The Medical Costs of Gunshot Injuries in the United States. *Journal of the American Medical Association* 282, no. 5 (August 4): 447–54.

Cook, Philip J., and James A. Leitzel. 1996. 'Perversity, Futility, Jeopardy': An Economic Analysis of the Attack on Gun Control. *Law and Contemporary Problems* 59 (1): 91–118.

Cook, Philip J., and Jens Ludwig. 1996. *Guns in America: Results of a Comprehensive Survey of Gun Ownership and Use*. Washington, D.C.: Police Foundation.

———. 1998. Defensive Gun Uses: New Evidence from a National Survey. *Journal of Quantitative Criminology* 14 (2): 111–31.

Cook, Philip J., Jens Ludwig, and David Hemenway. 1997. The Gun Debate's New Mythical Number: How Many Defensive Gun Uses per Year? *Journal of Policy Analysis and Management* 16: 463–69.

Cook, Philip J., S. Molliconi, and T. B. Cole. 1995. Regulating Gun Markets. *Journal of Criminal Law and Criminology* 86: 59–92.

Cork, Daniel. 1999. Examining Time-Space Interaction in City-Level Homicide Data: Crack Markets and the Diffusion of Guns Among Youth. *Journal of Quantitative Criminology* 15: 379–406.

Cullen, Julie Berry, and Steven D. Levitt. 1999. Crime, Urban Flight, and the Consequences for Cities. *Review of Economics and Statistics* 81 (2): 159–69.

Cummings, P., T. D. Koepsell, D. C. Grossman, J. Savarino, and R. S. Thompson. 1997. The Association between the Purchase of a Handgun and Homicide or Suicide. *American Journal of Public Health* 87: 974–78.

Cutler, David M., and Elizabeth Richardson. 1997. Measuring the Health of the U.S. Population. In *Brookings Papers on Economic Activity, Microeconomics*, 217–71. Washington, D.C.: Brookings Institution.

———. 1998. The Value of Health: 1970–1990. *American Economic Review* 88 (2): 97–100.

Davis, Y., J. L. Annest, K. E. Powell, and J. A. Mercy. 1996. An Evaluation of the National Electronic Injury Surveillance System for Use in Monitoring Nonfatal Firearm Injuries and Obtaining National Estimates. *Journal of Safety Research* 27: 83–91.

Dawson, Robert. 1992. An Empirical Study of Kent Style Juvenile Transfers to Criminal Court. *St. Mary's Journal* 23: 975.

Desvousges, William H., F. Reed Johnson, Richard W. Dunford, Kevin J. Boyle, Sara P. Hudson, and K. Nicole Wilson. 1993. Measuring Natural Resource Damages with Contingent Valuation: Tests of Validity and Reliability. In *Contingent Valuation: A Critical Assessment*, ed. Jerry A. Hausman, 91–164. Amsterdam: North Holland.

DeVivo, M. J. 1997. Causes and Costs of Spinal Cord Injury in the United States. *Spinal Cord* 35: 809–13.

Diamond, Peter A., and Jerry A. Hausman. 1993. On Contingent Valuation Measurement of Nonuse Values. In *Contingent Valuation: A Critical Assessment*, ed. Jerry A. Hausman, 3–38. Amsterdam: North Holland.

———. 1994. Contingent Valuation: Is Some Number Better than No Number? *Journal of Economic Perspectives* 8 (4): 45–64.

Donohue, John J., and Peter Siegelman. 1998. Allocating Resources among Prisons and Social Programs in the Battle against Crime. *Journal of Legal Studies* 27: 1–43.

Dvorak, Petula. 1999. D.C. Gun Buyback Drew Old, Cheap Guns, Analysis Finds. *Washington Post* (Washington, D.C.) December 16.

Dykstra, Robert R. 1968. *The Cattle Towns*. Lincoln: University of Nebraska Press.

Engen, Eric M., and William G. Gale. 1997. Consumption Taxes and Saving: The Role of Uncertainty in Tax Reform. *American Economic Review* 87 (2): 114–19.

Expectancy Data. 1999. *The Dollar Value of a Day: 1997 Dollar Valuation*. Shawnee Mission, Kans.: Expectancy Data.

Federal Bureau of Investigation. 1997. *Uniform Crime Reports for the United States 1996* Washington, D.C.: U.S. Department of Justice.

———. 1998. *Uniform Crime Reports for the United States 1997*. Washington, D.C.: U.S. Department of Justice.

Feinstein, Jonathan S. 1993. The Relationship Between Socioeconomic Status and Health: A Review of the Literature. *Milbank Quarterly* 71 (2): 279–322.

Finkler, S. A. 1982. The Distinction Between Cost and Charges. *Annals of Internal Medicine* 96: 102–9.

Firestone, David. 1999. After Shootings, Nation's Schools Add to Security. *New York Times*, August 13, A1.

Fox, James A. 1996. *Trends in Juvenile Violence: A Report to the United States Attorney General on Current and Future Rates of Juvenile Offending*. Boston, Mass.: Northeastern University Press.

Freeman, Myrick A. 1993. *The Measurement of Environmental and Resource Values: Theory and Methods*. Washington, D.C.: Resources for the Future.

Fronstin, Paul. 1998. Sources of Health Insurance and Characteristics of the Uninsured: Analysis of the March 1998 Current Population Survey. *Employee Benefit Research Institute (EBRI) Issue Brief Number 204*.

Galanter, Mark, and David Luban. 1993. Poetic Justice: Punitive Damages and Legal Pluralism. *American University Law Review* 42: 1393.

Gayer, Ted, James T. Hamilton, and W. Kip Viscusi. Forthcoming. Private Values of Risk Tradeoffs at Superfund Sites: Housing Market Evidence on Learning about Risk. *Review of Economics and Statistics*.

General Accounting Office. 1991. *Accidental Shootings: Many Deaths and Injuries Caused by Firearms Could be Prevented*. Washington, D.C.: General Accounting Office.

Glaeser, Edward L. 1995. Cities, Information, and Economic Growth. *Cityscape* 1 (1): 9–47.

Grogger, Jeff, and Mike Willis. 1998. The Introduction of Crack Cocaine and the Rise of Urban Crime Rates. National Bureau of Economic Research Working Paper No. 6353, Cambridge, Mass.: National Bureau of Economic Research.

GunCite. 2000. International Gun Fatality Rates. Available: <www.guncite.com/gun_control_gcgvintl.html>. Accessed January 24, 2000.

Halbfinger, David M. 1998. Where Fear Lingers: A Special Report. A Neighborhood Gives Peace a Wary Look. *New York Times*, May 18.

Hamermesh, David S. 1998. Crime and the Timing of Work. National Bureau of Economic Research Working Paper No. 6613, Cambridge, Mass.: National Bureau of Economic Research.

Hanemann, Michael, John Loomis, and Barbara Kanninen. 1991. Statistical Efficiency of Double-Bounded Dichotomous Choice Contingent Valuation. *American Journal of Agricultural Economics* 73 (4): 1255–63.

Hanemann, W. Michael. 1994. Valuing the Environment through Contingent Valuation. *Journal of Economic Perspectives* 8 (4): 19–43.

Harwood, Henrick, Douglas Fountain, and Gina Livermore. 1998. *The Economic Costs of Alcohol and Drug Abuse in the United States 1992*. Washington, D.C.: National Institute on Drug Abuse, National Institutes of Health, U.S Department of Health and Human Services.

Hausman, Jerry A. 1993b. *Contingent Valuation: A Critical Assessment*. Amsterdam: North Holland.

Hausman, Jerry A., Gregory K. Leonard, and Daniel McFadden. 1993a. Assessing Use Value Losses Caused by Natural Resource Injury. In *Contingent Valuation: A Critical Assessment*, ed. Jerry A. Hausman, 341–63. Amsterdam: North Holland.

Health Care Finance Association. 1999 Medical Cost Data. Available: <www.hcfa.gov/stats/pufiles.htm Washington, DC>. Accessed February 23, 1999.

Heinzerling, Lisa. 1998. Regulatory Costs of Mythic Proportions. *Yale Law Journal* 107 (May): 1981–2070.

Hemenway, David. 1997a. The Myth of Millions of Self-Defense Gun Uses: An Explanation of Extreme Overestimates. *Chance* 10: 6–10.

———. 1997b. Survey Research and Self-Defense Gun Use: An Explanation of Extreme Overestimates. *Journal of Criminal Law and Criminology* 87: 1430–45.

Hill, Jeffrey M. 1997. The Impact of Liberalized Concealed Weapon Statutes on Rates of Violent Crime. Senior thesis, Public Policy, Duke University.

Hodgkinson, Virginia A., Murray S. Weitzman, Eric A. Crutchfield, Aaron J. Heffron, and Arthur D. Kirsch. 1996. *Giving and Volunteering in the United States, 1996*. Washington, D.C.: Independent Sector.

Hodgson, T. A., and M. R. Meiners. 1979. Guidelines for Cost of Illness Studies in the Public Health Service. Unpublished Report, U.S. Public Health Services, Washington, D.C.

Hu, T. W., and F. Sandifer. 1981. Synthesis of Cost of Illness Methodology—Final Report. Unpublished Report, National Center for Health Statistics, Washington, D.C.

Ihlanfeldt, Keith R. 1995. "The Importance of the Central City to the Regional and National Economy." *Cityscape* 1 (2): 125–50.

Ikeda, Robin M., Rachel Gorwitz, Stephen P. James, Kenneth E. Powell, and James A. Mercy. 1997. *Fatal Firearm Injuries in the United States 1962–1994: Violence Surveillance Summary Series, No. 3*. Atlanta, Ga.: National Center for Injury Prevention and Control.

Institute of Medicine. 1981. *Cost of Environment-Related Health Effects: A Plan for Continuing Study*. Washington, D.C.: National Academy Press.

Jacobs, James B., and Kimberly A. Potter. 1999. Comprehensive Handgun Licensing and Registration: An Analysis and Critique of Brady II, Gun Control's Next (and Last?) Step. *Journal of Criminal Law and Criminology* 89 (1): 81–110.

Jamison, Kay Redfield. 1999. *Night Falls Fast: Understanding Suicide*. New York: Alfred A. Knopf.

Jana, Reene. 1998. Questions for Ozzy Osbourne. *New York Times Magazine*, June 28.

Janofsky, Michael. 1999. New Program in Richmond Is Credited for Getting Handguns Off the Street. *New York Times* February 10.

Johns Hopkins Center for Gun Policy. 1999. *Personalized Gun Technology: A Description of Existing Personalized Gun Technologies and Possible Applications of Existing Technologies to Firearms*. Baltimore, Md.: Johns Hopkins Center for Gun Policy and Research.

Kahneman, Daniel, and Jack L. Knetsch. 1992. Valuing Public Goods: The Purchase of Moral Satisfaction. *Journal of Environmental Economics and Management* 22: 57–70.

Kahneman, Daniel, and Amos Tversky. 1979. Prospect Theory: An Analysis of Decision Under Risk. *Econometrica* 47: 263–93.

Keil, Julian E., Susan E. Sutherland, Rebecca G. Knapp, and Herman A. Tyroler. 1992. Does Equal Socioeconomic Status in Black and White Men Mean Equal Risk of Mortality? *American Journal of Public Health* 82 (8): 1133–36.

Kellermann, Arthur L., Frederick P. Rivara, G. Somes, D. T. Reay, and J. Francisco. 1992. Suicide in the Home in Relation to Gun Ownership. *New England Journal of Medicine* 326: 467–72.

Kennedy, David M., Anne M. Piehl, and Anthony A. Braga. 1996. Youth Violence in Boston: Gun Markets, Serious Youth Offenders, and a Use-Reduction Strategy. *Law and Contemporary Problems* 59 (1): 147–83.

Kessler, Daniel P., and Steven D. Levitt. 1999. Using Sentence Enhancements to Distinguish Between Deterrence and Incapacitation. *Journal of Law and Economics* 42: 343–63.

Kleck, Gary. 1984. Handgun-Only Control: A Policy Disaster in the Making. In *Firearms and Violence: Issues of Public Policy*, ed. D. B. Kates Jr., 167–99. Cambridge, Mass.: Ballinger.

———. 1997. *Targeting Guns: Firearms and Their Control*. New York: Aldine de Gruyter.

Kleck, Gary, and M. Gertz. 1995. Armed Resistance to Crime: The Prevalence and Nature of Self-Defense with a Gun. *Journal of Criminal Law and Criminology* 86: 150–87.

Kleck, Gary, and K. McElrath. 1991. The Effects of Weaponry on Human Violence. *Social Forces* 69: 669–92.

Kuby, Alma M., Lauris Imhof, and Hee-Choon Shin. 1999. *Fall 1998 National Gun Policy Survey: Methodology Report*. Chicago: National Opinion Research Center.

Laband, David N., and John P. Sophocleus. 1992. An Estimate of Resource Expenditures on Transfer Activity in the United States. *Quarterly Journal of Economics* 108: 959–83.

Landefeld, J. Steven, and Eugene P. Seskin. 1982. The Economic Value of Life: Linking Theory to Practice. *American Journal of Public Health* 76 (6): 555–66.

LeClere, Felicia B., Richard G. Rogers, and Kimberly D. Peters. 1997. Ethnicity and Mortality in the United States: Individual and Community Correlates. *Social Forces* 76 (1): 169–98.

Leitzel, James A. 1998. Evasion and Public Policy: British and U.S. Firearm Regulation. *Policy Studies* 19 (2): 141–57.

Levitt, Steven D. 1996. The Effect of Prison Population Size on Crime Rates: Evidence from Prison Overcrowding Legislation. *Quarterly Journal of Economics*, 319–51.

———. 1997. Using Electoral Cycles in Police Hiring to Estimate the Effect of Police on Crime. *American Economic Review* 87 (3): 270–90.

Levitt, Steven D., and Sudhir Alladi Venkatesh. 2000. An Economic Analysis of a Drug-Selling Gang's Finances. Quarterly Journal of Economics (In press).

Lillie-Blanton, Marsha, Rose Marie Martinez, Barbara Lyons, and Diane Rowland. 1999. *Access to Health Care: Promises and Prospects for Low-Income Americans*. Washington, D.C.: Kaiser Commission on Medicaid and the Uninsured.

Lipscomb, Joseph, M. C. Weinstein, and G. W. Torrance. 1996. Time Preference. In *Cost-Effectiveness in Health and Medicine*, ed. M. R. Gold, J. E. Siegel, J. B. Russell, and M. C. Weinstein, 214–46. New York: Oxford University Press.

Loftin, Colin, David McDowall, Brian Wiersema, and Talbert Cottey. 1991. Effects of Restrictive Licensing of Handguns on Homicide and Suicide in the District of Columbia. *New England Journal of Medicine* 325: 1625–30.

Lott, John R., and David B. Mustard. 1997. Crime, Deterrence and Right-to-Carry Concealed Handguns. *Journal of Legal Studies* 16 (1): 1–68.

Ludwig, Jens. 1998. Concealed-Gun-Carrying Laws and Violent Crime: Evidence from State Panel Data. *International Review of Law and Economics* 18: 239–54.

Ludwig, Jens, and Philip J. Cook, 2000. Homicide and Suicide Rates

Associated with Implementation of the Brady Handgun Violence Prevention Act. *Journal of the American Medical Association* (In press).

Ludwig, Jens, Greg J. Duncan, and Paul Hirschfield. 2001. Urban Poverty and Juvenile Crime: Evidence from a Randomized Housing-Mobility Experiment. *Quarterly Journal of Economics* (In press).

Ludwig, Jens, Greg J. Duncan, and Joshua Pinkston. 1999. Neighborhood Effects on Earnings and Welfare Receipt. Working Paper Northwestern University/University, of Chicago Joint Center for Poverty Research, Chicago, IL.

Maddala, G. S. 1977. *Econometrics*. New York: McGraw-Hill.

Manning, Willard G. 1998. "The Logged Dependent Variable, Heteroscedasticity, and the Retransformation Problem." *Journal of Health Economics* 17: 283–95.

Manning, Willard G., Emmett B. Keeler, Joseph P. Newhouse, Elizabeth M. Sloss, and Jeffrey Wasserman. 1991. *The Costs of Poor Health Habits*. Cambridge, Mass. Harvard University Press.

Max, Wendy, and Dorothy P. Rice. 1993. Shooting in the Dark: Estimating the Cost of Firearm Injuries. *Health Affairs* 12: 171–85.

May, John, David Hemenway, Roger Oen, and Khalid Pitts. 1999. When Criminals Are Shot: A Survey of Washington D.C. Jail Detainees. Working Paper, Prison Health Services, Indianapolis, Ind.

McDowall, David, C. Loftin, and Brian Wiersema. 1992. A Comparative Study of the Preventative Effects of Mandatory Sentencing Laws for Gun Crimes. *Journal of Criminal Law and Criminology* 83: 378–94.

McDowall, David, Colin Loftin, and Brian Wiersema. 1995. Easing Concealed Firearms Laws: Effects in Three States. *Journal of Criminal Law and Criminology* 86: 193–206.

McGonigal, Michael D., John Cole, C. William Schwab, Donald R. Kauder, Michael F. Rotondo, and Peter B. Angood. 1993. Urban Firearm Deaths: A Five-Year Perspective. *Journal of Trauma* 35 (4): 532–36.

McLaughlin, Colleen R., Jack Daniel, Scott M. Riener, Dennis E Waite, Patricia N. Reams, Timothy F. Joost, Jeff L. Anderson, and Alfred S. Gervin. 1998. Factors Associated with Assault-Related Firearm Injuries in Male Adolescents. Working Paper, Virginia Department of Juvenile Justice, Richmond, Va.

Michael, Robert T., John H. Gagnon, Edward O. Laumann, and Gina Kolata. 1994. *Sex in America: A Definitive Survey*. Boston: Little, Brown.

Miller, Marjorie. 1999. Former Beatle George Harrison Survives Attack. *News & Observer* (Raleigh, N.C.) December 31, A2.

Miller, Matthew, and David Hemenway. 1999. The Relationship between Firearms and Suicide: A Review of the Literature. *Aggression and Violent Behavior* 4 (1): 59–75.

Miller, Ted R., and Mark A. Cohen. 1996. Costs. In *The Textbook of*

Penetrating Trauma, ed. R. R. Ivatury and C. G. Cayten, 49–59. Baltimore, Md.: Williams and Wilkins.

———. 1997. Costs of Gunshot and Cut/Stab Wounds in the United States, With Some Canadian Comparisons. *Accident Analysis and Prevention* 29 (3): 329–41.

Miller, Ted R., Diane C. Lestina, and Rebecca Spicer. 1998. Highway Crash Costs in the United States by Driver Age, Blood Alcohol Level, Victim Age, and Restraint Use. *Accident Analysis and Prevention* 30 (2): 137–50.

Miller, Ted R., S. Luchter, and P. Brinkman. 1989. Crash Costs and Safety Investment. *Accident Analysis and Prevention* 21: 303–15.

Miller, Ted R., Nancy Pindus, John B. Douglass, and Sheila B. Rossman. 1995. *Databook on Nonfatal Injury: Incidence, Costs, and Consequences*. Washington, D.C.: Urban Institute Press.

Mishan, E. J. 1971. Evaluation of Life and Limb: A Theoretical Approach. *Journal of Political Economy* 79 (4): 687–705.

Mitchell, Robert Cameron, and Richard T. Carson. 1989. *Using Surveys to Value Public Goods: The Contingent Valuation Method*. Washington, D.C.: Resources for the Future.

Montgomery, Paul L. 1980. Police Trace Tangled Path Leading to Lennon's Slaying at the Dakota. *New York Times*, December 10, A1.

Moore, Michael J., and W. Kip Viscusi. 1988a. Doubling the Estimated Value of Life: Results Using New Occupational Fatality Data. *Journal of Policy Analysis and Management* 7 (3): 476–90.

———. 1988b. The Quantity-Adjusted Value of Life. *Economic Inquiry* 26 (3): 369–88.

———. 1990a. Discounting Environmental Health Risks: New Evidence and Policy Implications. *Journal of Environmental Economics and Management* 18 (2): S51–62.

———. 1990b. Models for Estimating Discount Rates for Long-Term Health Risks Using Labor Market Data. *Journal of Risk and Uncertainty* 3 (4): 381–402.

Morrow, David J. 1999. Carolina Bank Robberies Show that Friendliness Carries a Price. *New York Times*, May 2, A1.

Moscicki, E. K. 1995. Epidemiology of Suicidal Behavior. *Suicide and Life Threatening Behavior* 25: 22–35.

MSNBC. 1999, August 24. D.C. Gun Buyback Program. Available: http://bbs.msnbc.com/bbs/msnbc-current/posts/cx/132420.asp.

Nader, Ralph. 1965. *Unsafe at Any Speed: The Designed-in Dangers of the American Automobile*. New York: Grossman.

National Center for Health Statistics. 1988. *Vital Statistics of the United States*. Vol. 2 *Mortality, Mortality Data 1968–87*. Atlanta, Ga.: National Center for Health Statistics.

———. 1999. National Mortality Followback Survey 1993. Mortality

Data Documentation Available: <ftp.cdc.gov/pub/Health_Statistics/ NCHS/Dataset_Documentation/NMFS/ Hyattsville, MD>.

National Highway Traffic Safety Administration. 1983. *The Economic Cost to Society of Motor Vehicle Accidents*. Washington, D.C.: U.S. Department of Transportation.

National Institutes of Health. 1999. Data on Cases and Costs of Emphysema Available:<www.nhlbi.nih.gov Washington, DC>.

National Rifle Association. 1999. Federal Gun Regulations Available: <www.nra.org Washington, DC>. Accessed December 17, 1999.

———. 2000. Project Exile Available: <www.nraila.org Washington, DC>. Accessed January 28 2000.

Neal, Derek A., and William R. Johnson. 1996. The Role of Premarket Factors in Black-White Wage Differences. *Journal of Political Economy* 104 (5): 869–95.

New York Times. 1999. Terror in Littleton: Guns in School Shootings Are Identified. *New York Times*, April 23, A15.

Noble, Christopher. 1999. Gun Makers Say Planned U.S. Lawsuit Makes No Sense. *Reuters*, December 8.

O'Connell, Vanessa. 1999. Swiss Company Will Be the First to Market a 'Smart Gun'. *Wall Street Journal*, December 13.

Office of Juvenile Justice and Delinquency Prevention. 1999. Promising Strategies to Reduce Gun Violence. Washington, D.C.: U.S. Department of Justice, Office of Juvenile Justice and Delinquency Prevention.

Pierce, Glenn L., and William J. Bowers. 1981. The Bartley-Fox Gun Law's Short-Term Impact on Crime in Boston. *Annals of the American Academy of Political and Social Science* 445: 120–37.

Portney, Paul R. 1981. Housing Prices, Health Effects, and Valuing Reductions in the Risk of Death. *Journal of Environmental Economics and Management* 8 (1): 72–78.

———. 1994. The Contingent Valuation Debate: Why Economists Should Care. *Journal of Economic Perspectives* 8 (4): 3–17.

Rennison, Callie Mae. 1999. *Criminal Victimization 1998: Changes 1997– 98 with Trends 1993–98. (NCJ 176353)*. Washington, D.C.: Bureau of Justice Statistics.

Reuter, Peter, Robert MacCoun, and P. Murphy. 1990. *Money from Crime: A Study of the Economics of Drug Dealing in Washington, D.C.* Santa Monica, Calif.: RAND.

Reuters. 2000. 'Smart Gun' Development Hampered by Money Woes. *Reuters*, January 4.

Revesz, Richard L. 1999. Environmental Regulation, Cost-Benefit Analysis, and the Discounting of Human Lives. *Columbia Law Review* 99 (4): 941–1017.

Rice, Dorothy P., and Ellen J. MacKenzie, and Associates. 1989. *Cost of Injury in the United States: A Report to Congress 1989*. San Francisco,

Calif.: Institute for Health & Aging, University of California; Injury Prevention Center, Johns Hopkins University.

Richmond Times-Dispatch. 1996. Newton's Law. Editorial. *Richmond Times-Dispatch* (Richmond, Va.), June 7, A16.

Roberts, R. R., P. W. Frutos, G. G. Ciavarella, L. M. Gussow, E. K. Mensah, L. M. Kampe, H. E. Straus, G. Joseph, and R. J. Rydman. 1999. Distribution of Variable vs. Fixed Costs of Hospital Care. *Journal of the American Medical Association* 281: 644–49.

Robuck-Mangum, Gail. 1997. Concealed Weapon Permit Holders in North Carolina: A Descriptive Study of Handgun-Carrying Behavior. M.Sc. Thesis, School of Public Health, University of North Carolina.

Rom, Mark C. 1997. *Fatal Extraction: The Story behind the Florida Dentist Accused of Infecting His Patients with HIV and Poisoning Public Health.* San Francisco: Jossey-Bass.

Rosen, Sherwin. 1986. The Theory of Equalizing Differences. In *The Handbook of Labor Economics*, ed. Orley Ashenfelter and Richard Layard, 641–92. Amsterdam: North Holland.

Roth, Jeffrey A., and Christopher S. Koper. 1997. *Impact Evaluation of the Public Safety and Recreational Firearms Use Protection Act of 1994.* Washington, D.C.: Urban Institute.

Rowland, Diane, Judith Feder, and Patricia Seliger Keenan. 1998. Uninsured in America: The Causes and Consequences. In *The Future U.S. Health Care System: Who Will Care for the Poor and Uninsured?* ed. Stuart H. Altman, Uwe E. Reinhardt, and Alexandra E. Shields, 25–44. Chicago: Health Administration Press.

Saltzman, L., J. A. Mercy, Patrick W. O'Carroll, M. L. Rosenberg, and P. H. Rhodes. 1992. Weapon Involvement and Injury Outcomes in Family and Intimate Assaults. *Journal of the American Medical Association* 267: 3043–47.

Schelling, Thomas C. 1968. The Life You Save May Be Your Own. In *Problems in Public Expenditure and Analysis*, ed. Samuel B. Chase, 127–62. Washington, D.C.: Brookings Institution.

Schiller, David. 1998. Project Exile. In Project Exile Available: *www.vahv.org/Exile/intro.htm*. Accessed January 16, 2000.

Schwab, C. William, et al. 1999. Urban Firearm Deaths: Trends over a Decade. Unpublished paper, University of Pennsylvania School of Medicine, Philadelphia.

Seattle Times. 1997. Pollution Triggers Asthma: Children are Most Vulnerable. *Seattle Times* August 3, B7.

Shavell, Steven. 1993. Contingent Valuation of the Nonuse Value of Natural Resources: Implications for Public Policy and the Liability System? In *Contingent Valuation: A Critical Assessment*, ed. Jerry A. Hausman, 371–88. Amsterdam: North Holland.

Sheley, Joseph F., and James D. Wright. 1993. *Gun Acquisition and Pos-*

session in Selected Juvenile Samples. Washington, D.C.: National Institute of Justice.

Sherman, Lawrence W., James W. Shaw, and Dennis P. Rogan. 1995. *The Kansas City Gun Experiment*. Washington, D.C.: National Institute of Justice.

Sink, Mindy. 1999. Shootings Intensity Interest in Home Schooling. *New York Times*, August 11, A18.

Smith, Tom W. 1997. A Call for a Truce in the DGU War. *Journal of Criminal Law and Criminology* 87 (4): 1462–69.

Smith, V. Kerry, and Carol Gilbert. 1984. The Implicit Risks to Life: A Comparative Analysis. *Economics Letters* 16: 393–99.

Sorlie, Paul D., Eric Backlund, and Jacob B. Keller. 1995. U.S. Mortality by Economic, Demographic, and Social Characteristics: The National Longitudinal Mortality Study. *American Journal of Public Health* 85 (7): 949–56.

Spitzer, Robert J. 1998. *The Politics of Gun Control*. New York: Chatham House.

Sudman, Seymour, and Norman Bradburn. 1974. *Response Effects in Surveys: A Review and Synthesis*. Chicago: Aldine.

Swetnam, George. 1980. *Andrew Carnegie*. Boston: Twayne Publishers.

Teret, Stephen P., Daniel W. Webster, and Jon S. Vernick, et al. 1998. Support for New Policies to Regulate Firearms: Results of Two National Surveys. *New England Journal of Medicine* 339 (12): 813–18.

Thomas, Emory. 1993. Attacks on Visitors Spur Downturn in Florida Tourism—Busy Season is Quiet as Foreign Travelers Turn to Other Destinations. *Wall Street Journal*, December 28, B6.

Tolley, George S., Donald S. Kenkel, and Robert G. Fabian. 1994. *Valuing Health for Policy: An Economic Approach*. Chicago: University of Chicago Press.

Torry, Saundra. 1999. Federal-Local Gun Control Venture Stymied by Success. *Washington Post*, September 11, A1.

U.S. Bureau of the Census. 1986. *Current Population Survey, March 1986, Tape Technical Documentation*. U.S. Department of Commerce, Bureau of the Census, Data User Services Division.

———. 1996. *Statistical Abstract of the United States, 1996*. Washington, D.C.: U.S. Government Printing Office.

———. 1997. *Statistical Abstract of the United States: 1997 (117th Edition)*. Washington, D.C.: U.S. Government Printing Office.

———. 1999a. *Statistical Abstract of the United States, 1999*. Washington, D.C.: U.S. Government Printing Office.

———. 1999b. State Population Estimates Available: *www.census.gov/ population/socdemo Washington, D.C.* Accessed February 22, 1999.

U.S. Office of Management and Budget. 1989. *Regulatory Program of the United States*. Washington, D.C.: U.S. Office of Management and Budget.

Van Dijk, Jan, and Pat Mayhew. 1993. Criminal Victimization in the Industrialized World: Key Findings of the 1989 and 1992 International Crime Surveys. In *Understanding Crime: Experiences of Crime and Crime Control*, ed. Anna Alvazzi del Frate, Ugljesa Zvekic, and Jan van Dijk. Rome: United Nations Interregional Crime and Justice Research Institute.

Vernick, Jon S., Z. F. Meisel, Stephen P. Teret, and S. W. Hargarten. 1999. "I Didn't Know the Gun Was Loaded": An Examination of Two Safety Devices That Can Reduce the Risk of Unintentional Firearm Injuries. *Journal of Public Health Policy* 20 (4): 427–40.

Virginians Against Handgun Violence. 2000. Project Exile. Available: *www.vahv.org/Exile/intro.htm Richmond, VA*. Accessed January 27, 2000.

Viscusi, W. Kip. 1993. The Value of Risks to Life and Health. *Journal of Economic Literature* 31 (4): 1912–46.

———. 1998. *Rational Risk Policy: The 1996 Arne Ryde Memorial Lectures*. New York: Oxford University Press.

Viscusi, W. Kip, and W. Evans. 1990. Utility Functions that Depend on Health Status: Estimates and Economic Implications. *American Economic Review* 80 (2): 353–74.

Viscusi, W. Kip, James T. Hamilton, and Ted Gayer. Forthcoming. Quantifying and Valuing Environmental Health Risks. In *The Handbook of Environmental Economics*. Elsevier, North Holland.

Viscusi, W. Kip, Wesley A. Magat, and Anne Forrest. 1988. Altruistic and Private Valuations of Risk Reduction. *Journal of Policy Analysis and Management* 7 (2): 227–45.

Viscusi, W. Kip, and Michael J. Moore. 1989. Rates of Time Preference and Valuations of the Duration of Life. *Journal of Public Economics* 38: 297–317.

Washington Post. 1999a. And the Guns Blaze On. Editorial. *Washington Post*, September 17.

———. 1999b. Handguns: Who Will Stand Up? Editorial. *Washington Post*, April 28.

Webster, D. W., and Mark K. Starnes. 1999. *Reexamining the Effects of Gun Storage Laws on Unintentional Firearm Deaths to Children*. Baltimore, Md.: Johns Hopkins Center for Gun Policy and Research.

Weil, Douglas. 1997. Traffic Stop: How the Brady Act Disrupts Interstate Gun Trafficking. Washington, D.C.: Center to Prevent Handgun Violence.

Weil, Douglas S., and Rebecca C. Knox. 1996. Effects of Limiting Handgun Purchases on Interstate Transfer of Firearms. *Journal of the American Medical Association* 275 (22): 1759–61.

Weisbrod, Burton A. 1961. *Economics of Public Health*. Philadelphia: University of Pennsylvania Press.

———. 1971. Costs and Benefits of Medical Research: A Case Study of Poliomyelitis. *Journal of Political Economy* 79: 527–44.

Welsh, Patrick. 1999. The Price of Protection. *U.S. News and World Report*, May 3, p. 28.

Wills, Garry. 1999. *A Necessary Evil: A History of American Distrust of Government*. New York: Simon and Schuster.

Wilson, James Q. 1995. Crime and Public Policy. In *Crime*, ed. James Q. Wilson and Joan Petersila, 489–507. San Francisco: Institute for Contemporary Studies.

Wilson, William Julius. 1987. *The Truly Disadvantaged*. Chicago: University of Chicago Press.

Wintemute, Garen J., Carrie A. Parham, James J. Beaumont, Mona A. Wright, and Christiana M. Drake. 1999. Mortality among Recent Purchasers of Handguns. *New England Journal of Medicine* 341 (21): November: 1583–89.

Wolfgang, Marvin E. 1958. *Patterns of Criminal Homicide*. Philadelphia: University of Pennsylvania Press.

Wright, James D., Peter H. Rossi, and K. Daly. 1983. *Under the Gun: Weapons, Crime and Violence in America*. Hawthorne, N.Y.: Adeline.

Wright, James D., and Peter H. Rossi. 1994. *Armed and Considered Dangerous: A Survey of Felons and Their Firearms (Expanded Edition)*. New York: Aldine de Gruyter.

Wright, Mona A., Garen J. Wintemute, and Frederick P. Rivara. 1999. Effectiveness of Denial of Handgun Purchase to Persons Believed to Be at High Risk for Firearm Violence. *American Journal of Public Health* 89 (1): 88–90.

Yates, F. 1981. *Sampling Methods for Censuses and Surveys*. 4th edition revised and enlarged. London: Charles Giffin.

Zeckhauser, Richard J., and Anthony C. Fisher. 1995. Averting Behavior and External Diseconomies. In *Environmental and Resource Economics: Selected Essays of Anthony C. Fisher*, ed. Anthony C. Fisher, 116–46. Brookfield, Vt.: Edward Elgar.

Zimring, Franklin E. 1968. Is Gun Control Likely to Reduce Violent Killings? *University of Chicago Law Review* 35: 21–37.

———. 1972. The Medium is the Message: Firearm Calibre as a Determinant of Death from Assault. *Journal of Legal Studies* 1: 97–124.

———. 1998. *American Youth Violence*. New York: Oxford University Press.

Zimring, Franklin E., and Gordon Hawkins. 1997. *Crime Is Not the Problem: Lethal Violence in America*. New York: Oxford University Press.

DATE DUE